T0349355

GOOD SEX

STORIES, SCIENCE, AND STRATEGIES
FOR SEXUAL LIBERATION

Candice Nicole Hargons, PhD

Row House Publishing recognizes that the power of
justice-centered storytelling isn't a phenomenon; it is essential for
progress. We believe in equity and activism, and that books—and
the culture around them—have the potential to transform the
universal conversation around what it means to be human.

Thank you for being an important part of the conversation
and holding sacred the critical work of our authors.

Library of Congress Cataloging-in-Publication Data
Available Upon Request

ISBN 978-1-955905-79-4 (HC)
ISBN 978-1-955905-80-0 (eBook)

Printed in the United States
Distributed by Simon & Schuster
First edition

10 9 8 7 6 5 4 3 2 1

To Tonja Marie Crowell

CONTENTS

What Is Good Sex
and Why You're Worthy of It

As a kid, my sex education was a hodgepodge of information from various random sources: the Encyclopedia Britannica my grandmother kept on her bookshelf, the garbage bag of porn VHS tapes my grandfather hid deep in the back of a closet, the Bible, Cosmopolitan magazines, the prototypical abstinence-only high school health teacher talk, '90s hip-hop, and pretending to be asleep so I could overhear the sexual escapades of my aunt Tonja as she braided and beaded my hair. I was constantly seeking sexual knowledge, but I was ill-informed. Talking about sex was not a conversation I felt I could initiate with my family members directly. Still, I was at least creative enough to synthesize what I learned, assert some ideas about what sex should be, and share with my friends throughout high school. I've been a sex educator for a long time.

As a quirky Black girl from small-town western New York, I listened to Lil' Kim and Lauryn Hill as much as Bush and Oasis. I was precocious in many ways, including sexually. I moved to an even smaller town in Virginia, when I was almost thirteen, soon after having my first peck on the lips.

Despite the lack of comprehensive sex education, I made my partnered sexual debut at age fourteen. From there, I quickly went from "I'm saving myself until marriage" to being "fast." My partner was a JNCO jeans-wearing white boy with shoulder-length brown hair. He played drums in a garage band.

When the redneck white boy and the Yankee Black girl got together publicly, audaciously holding hands to indicate how *official* we were, it remixed a Southern small-town cultural recipe. His ruddy white skin was a remarkable contrast to my deep brown, unambiguously Black complexion, politically and practically. In Franklin, Virginia, where a train track not at all subtly separated the Black and white sides of town, he didn't quite live on the white side, and I didn't quite live on the Black side. Before he and I were first introduced, my friend's boyfriend wanted to do a meetup at my house to see if we'd like each other. I later learned that, as a warning, her boyfriend had cautiously mentioned to him, "She's Black though . . ." He decided to come see me anyway.

Our sexual exploration began at thirteen when our first French kiss turned my normal breath into a world-rearranging guttural moan. In the year spanning those two time points, we sampled from the non-intercourse sexual behavior menu: passionate French kissing, writing erotic notes, sexy cordless phone calls, tentative and curious touching, sucking, rubbing, dry humping, fingering, licking. We eventually had intercourse when we were fourteen, a first for both of us. It wasn't as linear as first, second, and third base. And even though he got more orgasms out of the deal than I did, it was still good sex. It wouldn't have been good with just the sex acts; other ingredients like love, fun, and safety made it so.

Once my mom found a journal where we'd written notes to each other by surreptitiously passing the notebook back and forth through my little sister, and in it I talked about giving him head. In an attempt to mitigate harsher consequences for the unavoidable punishment, I tried assuring her it was all we'd done—it wasn't—and she was appalled.

"You mean you've been out here giving him all the pleasure and not getting anything for yourself?!"

This was one of the first messages I received about erotic equity from a family member. I love my mom for being a Black single parent of four who sustained the belief that she was pleasure-worthy. Cultural recipes had reiterated since at least the late '60s that Black women, especially, weren't deserving of sexual pleasure—shouldn't even be thinking of sex really—if they had to rely in any way on the government for financial support.

So, by the time I coordinated our sexual debut around my mom's travel for work, put on my cutest matching bra and panty set, lathered myself in Victoria's Secret's Strawberries and Champagne lotion, and invited him over to try what I thought, back then, was the holy grail of sex, it had been about a year of exploration. I felt excited, ready, and prepared. As a gentleman in our debut ritual, he took the risk to buy and bring condoms. We were "losing our virginity" together, another problematic sexual narrative, but it didn't feel like a loss to me. It felt like a monumental rite of passage.

I assumed the orgasm I effortlessly experienced through masturbation would come through penetration when a guy was involved. I'd experienced pleasure with him up until that point, but I had never come. Ever the optimist, I'd seen enough of the VHS porn tapes to believe the myth that not soon after his penis entered my vagina, I would be transported to vocal, orgasmic bliss.

Because we both had bought into the relationship recipe that penetrative sex is the best route to orgasm for males and females, I didn't have an orgasm, but he did. I faked it. I told him something silly about being a little sore, but satisfied, when we talked about it later that night. We had sex a few more times over the next month or so, then I dumped him for unrelated reasons. Still, looking back, I'm grateful that my sexual debut—the inaugural consensual sexual experience with a partner—had many of the good sex ingredients my research later examined: it was intimate, loving, consensual, and safe.

I didn't share an orgasmic experience with a partner until I was eighteen, but I did enjoy good sex in many other ways. In fact, I've had good sex most of my life, with my twenties and thirties being the decades where I reflected on the sexual recipes I'd learned and decided to challenge many of them. Black feminist scholars—Audre Lorde, Patricia Hill Collins, bell hooks, and Maya Angelou, to name a few— empowered me with the language and strategy to name, challenge, and change the recipes. As formidable resisters, they wrote about many of the ingredients shared in this book. Reading their work, I learned a lot, and I am still learning, about good sex.

GOOD SEX RECIPES AND INGREDIENTS

There are two sets of sexual ingredients: sexual behavior ingredients and sexual seasoning. Sexual behavior ingredients are a lot like foods in a meal: chicken, beef, fish, rice, etc. These are the action-based options one can choose from during sex (fingering, tribbing, masturbation, etc.). And then there are the seasonings that we use to enhance behavior. Just like chicken wings—all drummettes, fried hard please and thank you—can be spicy with buffalo sauce and sweet with honey BBQ, the same goes for sex. Oral sex can be romantic or raunchy, depending on the setting and dynamic between participants. There are certainly more sexual behaviors than I mentioned, as that isn't the scope of this book. This book features the societal influence, cultural background, and science behind sexual ingredients that enhance the experience of sexual behaviors.

Our personal sexual menus tend to be limited to popular culture trends, heteronormative science and medical findings, religious prescriptions, and what we pick up in passing. These become the recipes we cook from. It's where we get ideas about what good sex is, who gets to have it, and when it should happen. They also include, and are influenced by, the ways different forms of intersectional oppression (like racism, ageism, and heterosexism) trickle from the political culture into our sex lives. These ideas are like recipes for how we approach sex, as explained by sex researchers William Simon and John Gagnon. Their Sexual Scripting Theory introduced three levels of influence on our sexual lives and how we make sense of our sexual selves. Think of them as the three types of recipes:

- **Cultural Recipes:** These are the general ideas about good sex that come from our society, systems, and culture. Only certain people get to write these recipes, based on their privilege, and they distribute and withhold the good sex ingredients based on their corrupted sense of who is and is not worthy. Basically, all the isms start here, then trickle down to the . . .

- **Relationship Recipes:** These are the ways people act related to sex in relationship with others. The ingredients more readily offered from the cultural recipes are acted out here, as well as the things individuals truly desire or fantasize about in the . . .

- **Self-Recipes:** These are the personal beliefs, desires, fantasies, and expectations about good sex and the self. Because desires and fantasies are only minimally influenced by the other levels, some people who can resist social and structural pressure more than others keep their self-recipes relatively intact. These resisters show us the way if we're lucky enough to learn from them.

Sexual recipes, when influenced by oppression versus liberation, compromise (and sometimes eliminate) our ability to enjoy good sex. Basically, they under-season the chicken or put raisins in the potato salad. And it isn't a mistake. Sexual oppression has been intentionally constructed by religious, medical, educational, media, and political systems. Capitalism and classism can reduce sexual functioning. Racism and sexism can degrade sexual passion. Heterosexism, ageism, and ableism can deteriorate reciprocity. All the isms get in the way of intimate justice and erotic equity.

Intimate justice, according to Shatema Threadcraft, is focusing on fairness and care within our closest relationships as a critical site of liberation. In this case, sexual relationships. As a complementary lens to help us understand the origins of the many oppressions affecting our sexual selves, erotic equity, as defined by Sara McClelland, implicates the systems and structures that impact our access to the ingredients of good sex. Without them, sexual liberation is more likely a radical fantasy than a reality. Both intimate justice and erotic equity will be explained more in-depth in this chapter.

It's important to note that the story isn't as straightforward as *marginalization equals bad sex.* Some of us with multiple marginalized identities develop revolutionary outlooks on sexual liberation, benefiting from good sex more readily than people with privileged identities. For example, lesbians experience heterosexism and other oppressions, yet they report a higher percentage of orgasms during their most recent sexual experience than their heterosexual cis women peers. Queer women have something valuable to teach all of us about good sex and the erotic: word to Audre Lorde.

A surefire route to sexual liberation is exploring good sex ingredients with intention. This book will introduce you to some familiar and less familiar ingredients to good sex, or the sex that is good to and for you and whoever else is involved. With these ingredients, you can make your own recipes.

SHARING SEX SCIENCE

Finding out at twenty-five that being a sex researcher was an actual career option was such a delicious gift. Being a sex therapist was a way to help others experience sex that was good to and for them, so I pursued my master's degree in professional counseling. Then a mentor encouraged me to further my education by earning a PhD in counseling psychology. I'd taken all the sex-related classes my university offered. Learning how I could not only help others learn how to have good sex and realize sexual liberation, but I could also conduct the science of it . . . orgasmic yes!

When I started my tenure track job as an assistant professor, that's what I set out to do. I've coauthored over seventy research articles, many about sex and liberation. A year after the pandemic, my RISE[2] research team at the University of Kentucky and sexologists throughout the United States led the Big Sex Study.

If you could define good sex in three words, what would they be?

We asked over four hundred people with diverse ethnicities, ages, sexual and gender identities, and socioeconomic statuses this question and hundreds more in surveys, interviews, and focus groups from February 2021 to May 2022. The answers were as varied as their identities, but we distilled them down to a top twenty list: 1) Passionate; 2) Intimate; 3) Fun; 4) Pleasurable; 5) Satisfying; 6) Reciprocal; 7) Connected; 8) Consensual; 9) Orgasmic; 10) Nasty/ Kinky; 11) Exciting; 12) Liberating; 13) Loving; 14) Spiritual; 15) Sensual; 16) Communicative; 17) Wet; 18) Safe; 19) Relaxing; 20) Comfortable. The ingredients to good sex were selected from this list. Some were so foundational, like consent, that it couldn't be considered a seasoning. If good sex is a delicious meal you've created, you can't say you've created it if it wasn't consensual. Some were combined to make the meaning clearer. For example, gratifying was combined with satisfying.

Among the people we surveyed, the twenty ingredients of good sex were mostly similar, but they were ranked differently based on gender and sexual identity, which is important because good sex is not a set recipe. These ingredients are options that should be available and accessible to all of us. They can have greater or lesser importance depending on who we are, and that's okay. For example, for trans people who answered the "what is good sex" question, passion wasn't the top ranked, pleasure was. The world's violent treatment of trans folks in the past several decades gives us some insight into why they'd rank it differently. Pleasure as activism is a helpful antidote to extraordinary pain they've been subjected to. So, as you read this book, consider your identities and where your ingredients, recipes, and overall menu come from and what you want them to be.

THE UNSEASONED SEXUAL MENU

Imagine there's a sex menu, but instead of it being tailored to your unique desires and well-being, other people decide what recipes and ingredients you get to order. And the people are wealthy, white, heterosexual men from the sixteenth century. Some ingredients are good to and for you, but they're usually reserved for a tiny group of people. Some foundational figures in sex research push for erotic equity, or access to all the ingredients for everyone, but at every turn there is backlash preventing most people from even knowing some ingredients exist or are available to them.

Here are their most popular recipes today:

Jeff is a young, white American, heterosexual cisgender man. He's neurotypical, college educated, attractive, tall, slim, muscular, able-bodied, and Christian.

Jill, a white American, heterosexual cis woman, is also attractive, slim, neurotypical, college educated, and Christian.

The two have been marriage-bound since courtship, eager for a lifetime of vanilla, missionary, penis-in-vagina penetrative sex. They waited until marriage and have been, and will only be, sexual with each other until death.

According to standard, unseasoned Western world sex recipes, Jeff has earned—is entitled to—sexual pleasure frequently and enthusiastically from Jill by being a financial provider. He is to be stoic and strong, no matter what. He is always in leadership.

Jill wants children (and maybe some semblance of a care-focused career, but nothing too ambitious) and a comfortable life that her lesser esteemed and compensated profession cannot provide, so her sexual pleasure is optional. Still, she affirms that Jeff is an amazing lover whether he is or is not.

They are to have sex several times per week, or as often as Jeff desires it, because his desires are supreme. They are to have more than one child, as many as they can afford, and because they did things "the right way," they should never have to consider abortion. Every time they give birth, they immediately begin feeding their kids the same recipes they've been socialized in, so their kids one day follow the same sexual path.

This is an amalgamation of a bunch of cultural recipes most of us are force-fed regularly. A lot of pseudoscience went into the creation and maintenance of the unseasoned sexual menu, and it reinforces that these are the only people who deserve good sex. Whether or not you buy into it, these ideals offer currency by way of social capital, credibility, and value.

Simon and Gagnon suggest what we do sexually is shaped by the people we imagine upholding these recipes, even if they aren't there in the sexual space with us. For example, having sex with a certain number of people, or lying about the number of people you've had sex with, to align with the cultural recipe of purity as a valued attribute happens on the relationship level. Many people adopt the full unseasoned sexual menu wholesale, even if they don't have the interest, means, option, or access to do so. We see that on the self-recipe level.

Self-recipes allow you to identify how aligned your personal desires and behaviors are with cultural recipes. Do you desire sex with one person and only one person? What gratification, if any, does your sexual choice provide you? Could you see yourself as worthy of love, resources, and opportunities if you decided to have sex with ten people instead? What about one hundred? How does shame, disgust, pleasure, hope, and fear move in your body, influencing your sexual decisions and how you interpret the cultural recipes at large and the relationship recipes others act out?

It's important to know that the cultural recipes are just that: cultural. They are not static; they're informed by your race, class, gender, sexual identity, age, generation, body type, ethnicity, and region of the world, etc. Feel free to question *everything*. You need to do that for your sexual liberation; it's a key part of erotic equity.

Since the research of this book and the ingredients I present come from living in the United States as a Black woman, that lens will be central to all I say. My sample of research participants all identified as Black, even though they were diverse in ethnicity, gender, age, sexual identity, socioeconomic status, and body size. It's valuable to sit with how I wrote a book about good sex for people of all races when some of my theorizing comes from mostly Black participants. I make two cases for it. Nearly every other book I've read focusing exclusively on sex is written by someone white, yet those books are written as if they are universal and generalizable. Several of the components of those books still resonate with me, but the context of my history and daily life must be kept in mind to qualify which parts do and do not apply. I trust that readers of this book, with our various portfolios of privilege and marginalization, will be able to read it and resonate with it, take something of value from their reading, and share it with friends knowingly. And each reader will also have to consider where they've been left out or overlooked, whether intentionally or unintentionally. Where I likely do not know the context or applications that are most relevant for you based on your identities, you will fill in the gaps.

The research I cite, mine included, is often drawn from people with marginalized identities (women, people with disabilities, fat people, queer people, and people who experience multiple marginalizations), because perspectives can be more nuanced and clearer from the margins. Yet few sex books incorporate this essential scholarship. However, when I inevitably miss something that is relevant to your sexual menu-making, I invite you to trust your sense that what's missing is still worth knowing or considering. I hope it can be found in another book somewhere, and if it isn't in a book or text elsewhere, and writing is your thing, I hope you write it one day so I can cite it in another project.

The second case for the standpoint of this book, the Black wom-
anness of this subject, the intentionally chosen language, stories,
and science, is that the earliest sexual encounter on historical record
likely occurred with a Black woman. Dope, right!? The earliest modern human remains are from Omo Kibish I, a woman who lived in
Ethiopia over two hundred thousand years ago. To create most of us,
she too had to make her sexual debut. I often wonder what her ingredients were. Also, because of anti-Black racism, Black people have
been used as the avoidance benchmark for most sexual stereotypes in
the United States, and this is consequential for how the existing sexual
recipes are used and what new ingredients we need to adopt. In this
book, each ingredient is considered through the recipes of intimate
justice and erotic equity for the menu of sexual liberation.

Intimate justice, a liberation-driven cultural and relationship recipe, reminds us that our sexual and intimate relationships have been
too readily overlooked, despite being an essential site of liberation.
Everyone is worthy of good sex and sexual liberation, but people with
multiple marginalized identities have not been afforded this ascrip-
tion of inherent worthiness. In fact, most liberation movements have
largely ignored or pathologized the intimate and sexual equity, justice,
and freedom of people who operate outside of the dominant culture.
When we change recipes to include multiple ways of experiencing sex
and expressing sexualities, our systems must reconfigure the way they
work to uphold a human hierarchy.

Importantly, sexual liberation means you intentionally define and
express your sexual self in ways that are congruent with intimate justice, erotic equity, and your actual desires, needs, wants, and capacity.
For some people, this may still align with some of the existing cultural
recipes. Some seasonings may not work for you, and that can still be
good sex. You may want to wait until you're married to have sex, not
because you fear you won't be a moral, worthy human if you don't,

but because you have chosen that after careful self-reflection of what works for you. That's sexual liberation too.

Sexual liberation advocates for individual autonomy, not the rejection of all traditional sexual norms, but many people misunderstand this fact. By most accounts, I look like a traditional Black woman. I'm a monogamously married mom. I'm a cishet, middle-class, highly educated licensed counseling psychologist and professor. I'm neurotypical, able-bodied, and slim; I'm privileged in many ways. I've served on all kinds of psychology executive boards, won all kinds of research awards—all the trappings of elitist respectability organize my exterior world. But, at the core, I'm also a #HotGirl, a #HotGirlScientist if you will, of the "Cash Money Records taking over for the '99 and the 2000s" variety. In studying good sex, I try not to buy into any of the shit other people think gives me credibility as a researcher and expert, because the fact is: respectability politics won't save us. And it damn sure won't afford us sexual liberation.

To be clear, if you're not poly or kinky or anything else not on the traditional menu, good sex and sexual liberation aren't requiring that of you. It's simply asking you to critically consider why you're not and what you think it means for people who are. The goal is to practice good sex in a way that liberates you, not limits you to yet another set of recipes. Another goal is not trying to set the sexual menu for everyone else based on what you like, because minding your own business is free.

HOW TO READ *GOOD SEX*

The remaining chapters are a breakdown of each ingredient my research uncovered on the good sex list. As I noted, these ingredients of good sex are not, nor should they be, required for everyone. They should, however, be accessible to anyone who wants that type of seasoning in their sex life. Additionally, consent is essential no matter what. Think of each chapter as a mini lesson in that specific ingredient of good sex for you to read if that ingredient represents a part of your unique menu of sexual liberation. Read them all for pleasure or delve into the ones that resonate most deeply with you.

Each chapter begins with a story created from a fictionalized rendering of client and research participant stories from my work and a bit of background on the old recipes that influenced the enjoyment of that ingredient for better or worse, through the frameworks of intimate justice and erotic equity. Then I share some of the science related to that ingredient and strategies to season your sex life with it if you so choose. These are all based on over a decade of sex research and clinical work.

This book might introduce you to new ingredients you never realized were missing from your sex life. That's fantastic! Embrace your curiosity and be gentle with yourself as you explore. Remember, sexual liberation is a uniquely curated menu, not a microwave meal. It takes time to experiment and find the right ingredients to create sexual recipes that are good to and for you. Just like your taste buds change, your desires and needs will evolve too. And as some of the progress around equity, erotic and otherwise, is being targeted by several levels of government, standing for intimate justice will include remaking your sexual menu with political action alongside personal practice. So, whether you're sexually experienced or a neophyte, consider this book your invitation to get creative and courageous to cook up sex that is good to and for everyone involved!

Good Sex
is Intimate

Will and Malcolm had been dating seriously for about six months. Things seemed to be going well, until around the four-month mark. Malcolm wanted some space from the relationship, but instead of explaining his feelings, he just told Will they needed a break. This was a big change for Malcolm. With past boyfriends, he wouldn't say anything at all—he'd just stop texting them back, leaving them "on read." But Malcolm genuinely cared about Will and wanted to be more up-front. The truth was, the growing intimacy was overwhelming for him. He had been more open with Will than he had with anyone, and even during their sexual experiences he could tell Will really *knew* him. It felt good but also unsettling and unfamiliar, so he blurted out the break request without realizing Will might agree.

"It was weird, right? For me to be checking his social media every five minutes when I was the one who told him I needed the break." Malcolm, a short, brown-skinned Black man, chuckled nervously, pushing his shoulder-length black locs behind his ears. "I mean, I was good for like the first month or so. I was having me a little hot boy summer, figuring he would reach back out to me like the other guys had, once I'd not so subtly ghosted them." He tucked his left leg under his butt and looked over at Will. "But then he had the nerve to be unbothered, leaving me all the way alone. It stirred something in me. I realized I didn't actually *want* to take a break, I just needed some breathing room."

Will, a petite Korean American man, returned his gaze and grazed Malcolm's pinky with his own. "I was part respecting the boundary he'd asked for and part not even mad about the break because I also wasn't getting what I needed in the relationship, emotionally or sexually. They're connected to me. But I was glad he reached back out and asked me if I wanted to try this little therapy situation with him. I figured we could stand to talk about some things with someone."

Will was an anchor. According to *Wired for Love* author Stan Tatkin, as a securely attached person, Will sought closeness with Malcolm, was minimally insecure about the possibility that Malcolm might one day leave him, and was mostly open and communicative when his feelings began to grow. Anchors usually find each other, but this time Will found an island, someone with a more avoidant attachment style. Malcolm was struggling to reconcile his deep desire for closeness with his trepidation that closeness would become smothering, requiring more of him than he had to offer.

They had good sex in the beginning, but as the relationship revealed their typical patterns of relating, the good sex waned. Will realized Malcolm's need for distance, paired with his avoidance of healthy conflict, was getting in the way of the type of intimacy that kept him aroused. Research shows that intimacy and attachment are related to good sex in a few ways I'll address in the Science of Intimacy and Attachment section. This played out for Will and Malcolm, and it brought them into therapy.

Sex without a certain level of intimacy was a turn-off for Will. And sex with too much intimacy felt predictable and boring to Malcolm. They could both agree that they had the skills to please each other, but their relationship dynamics started to impact their sexual desire and satisfaction. Malcolm began to be less available and responsive to Will's invitations to spend time together. As an island, the alone time gave him a moment to self-regulate. He could then go back to Will feeling whole again. Our therapy work was to explain this need to both and honor the process of how islands and anchors operate. As an anchor, Will was less prone to chasing partners than what Tatkin calls a wave, or an anxiously attached person, might have been. That is, Will didn't feel abandoned and fearful that the relationship would end and never be repaired by Malcolm's need for space. He wasn't going to act out or chase Malcolm until he returned, but he was aware of his desires and used therapy to express them honestly. He let Malcolm know that he was prepared to honor his need for space, but when he had the energy and sense of wholeness to return, he needed him to come back with effort related to intimacy: a romance ritual.

CLOSENESS AND CONSENSUAL VULNERABILITY

Early definitions of *intimate* from the 1600s include sentiments such as "very familiar, innermost, or closely acquainted." In the 1990's, G.M. Timmerman defined *intimacy* as "a quality of a relationship in which the individuals must have reciprocal feelings of trust and emotional closeness toward each other and are able to openly communicate thoughts and feelings with each other. The conditions that must be met for intimacy to occur include reciprocity of trust, emotional closeness, and self-disclosure." Importantly, the researcher drew from many studies to develop this definition, and physical intimacy remained mostly separate. That means this definition of intimacy is a component of good sex, rather than good sex itself. Vulnerability is often a key component in the existing definitions of intimacy, and researchers are now clearer that empowered, consensual vulnerability met with affirming reinforcement is the process by which intimacy grows in many relationships.

Cultural recipes for intimacy are often grounded in patriarchy and misogyny. Intimacy has been feminized, such that attending to another person in a way that allows you to know them and receive their disclosures is stereotypically located in women and feminine of center peoples' purview. To be known well then becomes a privileged real estate afforded to the people women and feminine of center people are in relationship with, sometimes without the actuality or expectation of reciprocity. To be vulnerable, however, risks being a target for exploitation, invalidation, or even violence. The balance is incredibly complicated.

People with various forms of marginalized identities may also recognize this phenomenon: we know a lot more about the dominant cultures than they know about us. Disabled people often have to navigate buildings and entryways made for people who are able-bodied, so they are constantly receiving information about able-bodied people and what they value. Able-bodied people do not have to learn about disabled people in the same way. Similar to this, sexual partners often don't have the same level of privilege. This means their experiences with sex and intimacy are shaped by different expectations. One partner might be expected to take the lead in learning about the other's desires, which can be a lot of work that often goes unnoticed. But when we position intimacy as a power-down position, we miss an opportunity to be in a balanced relationship. Some songs and cultural recipes even frame intimacy as a communicable disease: people talk about "catching feelings" for someone as something to be avoided in the same way you'd avoid the flu.

To realize erotic equity in your sexual relationship, empathy, attention, and vulnerability are essential to intimacy and should be offered and received fairly. If one partner has not been required to cultivate the skill of being intimate, they will need to practice being vulnerable and responding positively to their partner's vulnerability. In contexts where intimacy is affirmed or rewarded, it is more likely to grow. It won't change overnight, but there are ways to develop empathy as a skill.

TYPES OF INTIMACY

Sexologist Shamyra Howard's book, *Use Your Mouth*, identifies seven types of intimacy: emotional, social, financial, spiritual, intellectual, physical, and sexual. Since the word *intimacy* is often used as a euphemism for sex, it makes sense that most people don't realize sexual intimacy is just one of many types. Howard explains that each type of intimacy offers a different path to a deeper connection, so they require unique approaches to nurture them. We tend to have preferences for one or two types of intimacy, but all of them can be beneficial. And each of the nonsexual intimacies can contribute to good sex. Brief definitions of each intimacy are:

- **Emotional Intimacy:** Sharing deep feelings, moods, vulnerabilities, and empathizing with another person, fostering a sense of trust and emotional connection.

- **Social Intimacy:** Enjoying shared activities, hobbies, and interests with someone, building a sense of companionship and belonging.

- **Financial Intimacy:** Communicating openly about finances, creating shared goals and a sense of trust around money matters.

- **Spiritual Intimacy:** Sharing spiritual or religious practices, beliefs, and values, and finding a sense of purpose and life meaning together.

- **Intellectual Intimacy:** Stimulating conversations, sharing ideas, and learning from and with each other, fostering a sense of mental connection and mutual respect.

- **Physical Intimacy:** Engaging in nonsexual forms of physical closeness, such as cuddling, holding hands, or expressing affection through other forms of nongenital or erogenous touch.

- **Sexual Intimacy:** Engaging in sexual forms of physical closeness through genital or erogenous touch.

SCIENCE OF INTIMACY AND ATTACHMENT

Attachment theories suggest most people are born motivated to seek closeness to caretakers and significant others for protection and nurturing. However, when people grow up in family systems that are emotionally neglectful or volatile, they're more likely to develop an insecure attachment style that becomes a barrier to their ability to experience many forms of intimacy. They may fear closeness and respond by pushing others away (avoidant attachment) or fear rejection of their need for closeness and try controlling others to get them to stay (anxious attachment). True to misogyny, the early days of attachment theory blamed this on the mother almost exclusively; however, newer and evolved theories underscore the family system, not simply one parent, as the unit in which attachment styles are formed. More modern theories on attachment offer a developmental model, where the evolution of one's attachment patterns are broken down by age (see Patricia Crittenden's dynamic-maturational model of attachment and adaptation, or DMM). However, for simplicity, the three types originally created by John Bowlby and contemporized by Stan Tatkin's model are shared here.

Romantic and/or sexual partners can buffer some of the distress experienced by insecurely attached partners. For avoidantly attached partners – islands - who may avoid intimacy more readily, having a partner who respects their autonomy validates how they see the world, and it acknowledges their good qualities without expressing a lot of emotion, which helps them after a conflict and when they feel insecure. For anxiously attached partners – waves - who deeply crave closeness, having an accommodating partner who avoids exacerbating conflict by retaliating and who demonstrates commitment to maintaining the relationship goes a long way.

In research by Jardin Dogan-Dixon and my research team, we examined how Black college students understand and navigate intimacy in their sexual relationships, discovering they perceive internal and external barriers to nonsexual intimacy. This, in turn, affects the quality of their sexual experience. People interviewed in the study mentioned several factors that hindered their ability to experience nonsexual intimacy. These included toxic narratives from family, friends, and the media. So, although they were having sex, and perhaps experiencing sexual intimacy, the other types of intimacy identified by Shamyra Howard felt lacking. Internal barriers to intimacy included maintaining limited or halting communication with sexual partners when it appeared they were developing closeness, focusing only on the casualness of the sex, and ending the relationships that were more intimate than they desired. These choices were similar to how Malcolm had engaged Will.

For Will, emotional intimacy was his key ingredient to good sex. Expressing emotions, being heard and validated, and perceiving one's partner is willing to share emotions are core to emotional intimacy.

Initially, Malcolm would disregard Will's emotions, minimizing them the way his had been minimized throughout his life by parents who were disgusted that their only son was gay from an early age. His emotions represented effeminacy to his parents, so they believed minimizing his emotional expression would make him more of a man. Malcolm didn't even realize his emotions had been minimized, because even though it didn't feel good, it was so normal. In turn, it was normal for him to do the same to Will. He had a hard time holding space for vulnerability, for himself and his partner, which felt unfulfilling for Will emotionally and sexually.

Esther Perel, a relationship therapist and author of *Mating in Captivity*, noted that, as it relates to good sex, intimacy is part trap, part embrace. Intimacy's complicated nature influences why relationship satisfaction increases as intimacy grows for some people and decreases for others. So, there is a bell curve in how intimacy becomes a part of good sex. With too much intimacy, the familiarity of the person may reduce their sexual appeal, especially if they struggle to establish their own sense of self. With too little intimacy, there may not be enough safety to enjoy sex deeply, especially if the person is experiencing various forms of marginalization.

STRATEGIES FOR INTIMATE GOOD SEX

Romance is a vulnerable act that can cultivate various forms of intimacy. The person initiating the romantic gesture is investing in making their partner feel seen and cared for. For people with anxious or avoidant attachments, any form of vulnerability can be difficult to express due to fear it won't be returned or it will be overused. Romance is a form of reverence, and doing it well requires an intimate attentiveness.

In addition to attachment style, intimate attentiveness is also related to one's mental health. For example, someone with ADHD might find it harder to maintain attention on their partner after the initial honeymoon phase (hyperfocus) wears off. Additionally, people who experience multiple forms of marginalization (discrimination based on overlapping social identities) often face a double burden. Their mental and emotional energy gets drained by constantly navigating systems of oppression. By the time they return home to their partner, they might be too depleted to fully engage. Even though they desire intimacy and closeness, they simply lack the energy for it. This often creates a bigger problem for women and feminine of center people. Society often judges us based on our ability to be attentive to others' needs. We're socialized to excel at caregiving and emotional labor. Meanwhile, men are frequently discouraged from expressing the same level of intimacy, thanks to patriarchal norms and misogyny. These cultural recipes prevent all of us from intentionally using intimacy as an ingredient. Instead, it gets used unskillfully or out of obligation.

This doesn't mean men and masculine-of-center individuals aren't interested in intimacy. In fact, they often desire it. However, they might need to actively develop those skills as adults since societal expectations during their childhood may not have encouraged them. In relationships, it's not the sole responsibility of their female or more feminine of center partners to teach them these skills. Even with the option of each partner buffering the other based on their attachment styles, cultivating intimacy is a personal journey. Seeking professional help can benefit people who have more barriers to intimacy and their partners.

That was the case with Malcolm and Will. Since Malcolm and Will came in for couples counseling, we focused some portion of the session on Malcolm's ability to offer emotional intimacy and Will's ability to buffer. Given the power dynamics in their relationship, with Malcolm as the more stereotypically masculine partner, the educational component was heavier on Malcolm. I provided activities, questions, and resources related to better understanding his attachment style and practicing various types of intimacy, especially emotional, that he could move through at his own pace. We were also able to use the therapy space to check back in and for Will to indicate how he'd observed Malcolm's willingness and capacity to change. Because Will was an anchor, he was open to buffering Malcolm's more avoidant tendencies if he knew Malcolm was invested in their relationship growth. As a result of the increased romance, as well as the respect for space, Malcolm and Will were able to improve their intimacy and enrich their experiences of good sex with each other.

Sexologist Shamyra offers several suggestions in her workbook, and I'll share a few here. If you are ready to cultivate intellectual intimacy, you can ask your partner to identify their three favorite topics to discuss. Then you can choose one or two to learn more about together and discuss. The romance rituals you and your partner develop should be undergirded by forms of intimacy you enjoy. Exploring romance in the ways that arouse you creates the safety and sense of vulnerability to enrich good sex.

For Will and Malcolm, they practiced intellectual and emotional intimacy most. As a sapiosexual, or someone who finds intelligence attractive and arousing, talking nerdy to Malcolm or being able to teach him something he wanted to learn turned him on. Cultivating intellectual intimacy by reading books together was his idea of romance. Also, as someone who needed emotional intimacy to make the sex good, the suggestion that they go to therapy together was an important olive branch for Will.

Which of the seven types of intimacies are priority for you? I suggest you rank them and start by cultivating only one. When you try to do too much too soon, you risk being overwhelmed. To better understand yourself as a human being with intimacy needs, divest from the idea that you don't have vulnerabilities or needs (or that having them makes you weak or shameful), and then communicate them with your sexual partner(s). A lot of people assume that cultivating intimacy is only for people in committed, romantic relationships, which is likely a function of the "avoid catching feelings" mindset, because intimacy can be cultivated among family, friends (even those with benefits), fuck buddies, one-night stands, and lifelong loves, all the same.

Also, consider your attachment style: are you a wave (anxious attachment), an island (avoidant attachment), or an anchor (secure attachment)? See *Wired for Love*, which will provide insight into your typical disposition toward intimacy. All the attachment styles are able to cultivate intimacy, but you may have an easier or harder time. That's okay. Sharing your attachment style with your partner also helps them better understand how you approach intimacy. It may allow them to appreciate the new practices you're trying together to cultivate a more intimate sex life.

Once Malcolm and Will were introduced to language to understand their attachment styles and each other's, they could call attention to when the need to be an island started to resurface for Malcolm. Malcolm learned to say that he was going to take a few days of space, not an indefinite amount of time, and when he returned, he was able to process what it was like for him and attend to the ways Will desired to be known. For Will, it was emotional intimacy, so having Malcolm there to empathize with him, rather than minimize, helped him feel a deeper sense of closeness.

Because they were committed to their long-term relationship, Malcolm began to see how the feelings of safety Will was creating for them both were still an act of emotional labor. He expressed more compassion and gratitude for Will's willingness to do that labor more as he developed the skill of it. In turn, they found that their sex life improved. Will was more into the sex because he felt more heard, seen, and valued by Malcolm. Malcolm felt less bored and restless with their sex because he saw Will's increased enthusiasm as incentive for his effort to grow his intimacy muscle. They had a better command of how to use the sexual skills they came in with in a more attuned way, listening for the small shifts in breathing and movements in their bodies during sex to increase their sense of closeness. For them, erotic equity wasn't each person doing the same thing. It was giving similar levels of effort to cultivate the intimacy that made the sex good. They both shared that even after tough therapy sessions, the sex was better for them because their sense of closeness was enhanced.

— 2 —

Good Sex
is Fun

Nakita and Joi had been together for three years, and they managed to hold on to their new relationship energy longer than most people. Whereas most people experience the normal shift out of that chemically induced phase between six to eighteen months, theirs lasted around two years. Because Nakita and Joi prioritized fun, albeit different types of fun, they were both surprised to hear that the honeymoon phase ending didn't mean something was wrong. Nakita and Joi acknowledged that their initial definition of fun might need to evolve. They came to therapy because they were interested in exploring new ways to keep their sex life fun in the long term. They started by giving me an example of a fun sexual experience.

"I told Nakita that I wanted a threesome with a guy for my birthday, and she was like, 'What kind of guys do you like?' So I named all these qualities: open-minded, generous, flexible, fine. She waited for me to finish the checklist and then asked straight up about size." Joi, a slim, Dominican, light-skinned cisgender woman, smiled as she told the story.

"I will preface this by saying I am not a woman that judges men on their size." Joi leaned in to convince me, and a shoulder-length auburn curl swung forward like a trapeze.

Nakita, a larger-bodied, Black American masculine-of-center woman interrupted, "So we're lying? Okay, that's fine. Okay."

Both women threw their heads back, erupting in laughter. A solid minute of laughter, with tears running down Nakita's almond cheeks, drew me into the moment with them. I didn't know where the story was going, but I was deeply invested.

Nakita chimed in, "I mean, we don't get organic dick often, so if we were planning to get some for her birthday, it should be dick worth getting. But she always picks a big strap with me."

Joi continued the story. "Anyways, we hit my friend Manny up. We've never had sex before, but he's always been fine, and I've always been curious about him. It's good to have a partner who is willing to have a little fun with you, so I am really grateful to Nakita for that. Manny was game! I didn't even have a chance to get the words all the way out before he told me he was about to hop in the shower. So Nakita and I were playing around the house, with the music bumping, drinks flowing, smoke blowing. Gir . . . ," she paused, slightly embarrassed, "I mean Dr. Hargons."

"Naw, girl is fine with me. It's a term of endearment."

"Right, right! So, girl, he gets there and starts partaking in the drinks. We're dancing the merengue, laughing, singing, then the bachata, touching, caressing. Clothes are gradually coming off. He's down to the boxer briefs. At this point, I'm read . . . dy. Nakita has unwrapped me like I'm the present, and she's stroking my hair, holding my head while he goes down on me. Birthday is birthday-ing. Then he says, 'You want your birthday present now?' To me, dick is never a present, and I was right again."

"So, overall, it was fun or . . . ?" I asked, confused about the ending.

"Yes, it was some of the most fun we've ever had. I came in his mouth, the penetration helped him get off, and then I strapped up and took Nakita over the edge. He was basically taking notes, like 'Damn, that's how y'all get it?' It wasn't weird either. I think he will be a better lover with what he is packing after seeing what can be done with fingers and a strap. Sometimes straight guys from my culture think the sex starts and ends with a dick. Like I said, I'm not a size ho, but you gotta know what you're doing with what you got. I got to enjoy dancing, laughter, head, and quality time with two really good people on my thirtieth birthday. It was the best type of fun."

Nakita added, "I loved it too. We literally spent no money. We were broke as fuck, but we had a time." Something about that joy radiated between them, such that just retelling the story set them aglow. They wanted to learn how they could keep that same joy and fun.

FOOLISHNESS OR FUN

Access to certain types of fun, and even how fun is defined, can be tied to economic and other types of privilege. Interestingly, however, examining the etymology of the word *fun*, we can see its earlier uses cast people who had fun as fools. This may have implications for good sex. Many of us fear being the butt of the joke at such a vulnerable time as sexual experiences. Yet being able to laugh at yourself and with your partner during sex ensures that you're teachable and willing to grow as a sexual being. Had Manny been afraid to learn from Joi and Nakita, letting machismo get in the way of being able to take himself less seriously, he would have missed out on a social, sensual, and achievement type of fun with them. For Nakita and Joi, prioritizing sensual and other types of fun had been a great benefit to their sex life for years.

Some people, particularly those who were parentified children or were socialized in strict stoicism by way of family, community culture, or work, may place less value on fun, let alone fun sex. It's important to examine the origins of our beliefs that equate "fun" with foolishness, particularly in the context of sexual experiences. This perspective might be hindering our ability to fully embrace joy, laughter, and other forms of fun during sex. Why do some people feel apprehension about being perceived as unserious during sex? What cultural or personal recipes have led us to associate seriousness with sex, potentially at the expense of enjoyment?

TOXIC SERIOUSNESS AND FORGOING FUN

Cultural recipes about being serious, or taken seriously, get conflated with maturity. They are also born of privileging rationality over frivolity. But it's possible to take life seriously, meaning really care about life, without being dragged into toxic seriousness that stifles our ability to experience sexual fun. Caroline Leaf, a Christian writer, first introduced the term *toxic seriousness* and reflected on the way fun and laughter are medicinal; they reduce our distress. Similarly, for a sexual experience to be good to you and for you, fun can serve as an important ingredient. Fun sex can be especially important for folks dealing with sexual problems or infertility. When you're focused on a specific outcome, like getting pregnant or keeping an erection, sex can get mechanical and boring. You might feel stuck doing the same things over and over, even if it "works." That drains all the fun out of it. For Joi and Nakita, their goal wasn't pregnancy. It was enriching an already good sex life. But as novelty wears off, getting stuck doing what has worked before can still manifest.

Some people have sex out of duty, rather than for fun and enjoyment. It is an obligation to which they've agreed, another type of contracted work or labor. They associate their sense of goodness and self-image with sexual frequency—a good wife has sex with her husband as often as he wants, or, to prevent a partner from cheating, you must meet all their sexual needs. This obligatory approach to sex can suck the fun out of it quickly.

Have you ever felt like you can't have fun freely? For many of us, especially people in marginalized groups, showing happiness can sometimes feel like a tightrope walk. We laugh a little too loud, maybe cheer a bit too hard, and suddenly it's a problem. Take the story of the Sistahs on the Reading Edge Book Club. These Black women were kicked off a wine train in 2015, all because they were having a good time and laughing together. It's crazy to think that celebrating a win, a graduation, or even just enjoying a night out can be seen as disruptive or even threatening. Think about it: when a mostly white college team wins, fans go wild! They might even burn a couch or two. But that's seen as good-natured excitement. Meanwhile, Black graduates expressing their joy at commencement might get their diplomas held hostage because their happiness is seen as "out of line." This double standard is frustrating. It's like our joy is a threat to someone. And awareness of this in everyday life can influence the way you have sexual fun, because you get so used to self-policing fun that nowhere feels like an allowable fun space.

But when you consider divesting from respectability politics as one way we can work to realize sexual liberation, isn't it beautiful that we can use joy as disruption, rather than over relying on anger? Fun can be a surprisingly powerful tool. It feels good, it's contagious (in a good way!), and it can be a great way to challenge the status quo, including sexual and other forms of oppression. Your vagina queefs during a certain position, and instead of your partner looking at you in disgust, you both laugh and figure out how that happens together. Your penis gets soft when you try to put the condom on, and instead of being shamed by your partner, you both laugh and go back to kissing, touching, and enjoying nonpenetrative sex.

THRILL FUN AND CHILL FUN

Very little research examines fun and sex together, so making sense of how they are related required understanding fun in general and drawing on my work with clients who struggled in this area. Psychologists I.C. McManus and Adrian Furnham aptly indicated that people mean different things when they use the word *fun*. Their study found that based on a survey of 1,100 people, sensual fun was one of five types:

- **Sensual:** Fun associated with romance, intimacy, and sex.

- **Sociability:** Fun enjoyed with others.

- **Contentment:** Fun associated with relaxation and peace.

- **Achievement:** Fun associated with challenges and accomplishment.

- **Ecstatic:** Fun associated with exhilaration and excitement.

Sex scientists haven't figured out yet if there's one "best" kind of fun for a good sex life, but they did find some interesting connections! People who are outgoing and adventurous (high in extraversion) tend to enjoy more sensual fun. On the other hand, folks who are super organized and rule followers (high in conscientiousness and agreeableness) might be less into it.

They also found five attitudes toward fun: fun requires risk-taking, fun requires fun people, fun is necessary for happiness, fun requires money, and fun requires spontaneity. All but the "fun is necessary for happiness" attitude were related to sensual fun, but the "fun requires money" attitude was the most highly correlated. That means the stronger someone believed in money being required for fun, the more likely they were to enjoy sensual fun.

Given what their study found, fun is a complex word that can describe an activity or a person, and there are a range of attitudes about fun. As was previously stated, what makes a sexual experience fun will differ based on your unique definition of fun. In addition to the five types of fun McManus and Furnham found, Harry Reis and colleagues break fun down into two simpler types: high activation pleasant and low activation pleasant. Let's call these types thrill fun and chill fun.

Thrill fun, or the kind of fun experienced with high arousal/activation, can facilitate feelings like excitement, amusement, enthusiasm, and other more alert moods. Chill fun, or the kind experienced with low arousal/activation, can create feelings like gratitude, calm, and relaxation. Both are positive and foster enjoyment, but in different ways. Of McManus's five types of fun, sensual, social, and achievement can be either a thrill or chill version, whereas the contentment type of fun would align with chill fun and ecstatic type of fun would align with thrill fun. Considering sensual fun, which includes sexual fun and other sensory enjoyments, thrill and chill are options for that too. For thrill fun sex, there might be adventure, exploration, and energetic movement. A sense of novelty can lead to thrill fun sex. For chill fun sex, there might be laughter, sensual dance, and less vigorous play. Depending on your tendency to shrink from or actively pursue fun, you may prefer one or the other more.

Reis's study also suggests "it ain't no fun if the homies can't have none," but not quite in the way Snoop Dogg suggested. Their study was related to game play, not sex, but the results may be somewhat transferable. There isn't anything wrong with solo sex, but when asked about peak pleasure, Shemeka Thorpe's work found Black women included partnered sex as an important element. Perhaps that's true for others, and maybe partnered sex would be rated more fun.

STRATEGIES FOR FREEING YOUR SEXUAL FUN

What experiences constitute fun for you? What were the benefits and consequences of fun at various times in your life? What messages have you received about your ability to have fun, especially in the context of a sexual experience? Answering these questions may help you better understand how you came to be more or less open to fun experiences. The associations we make to having fun, publicly and privately, give us access points to whether we include it in our sex lives.

Can you recall the most fun sexual experience of your life? The recollection exercise I facilitated with Nakita and Joi helped them both recognize the elements that they can readily include in their more recent sexual experiences. For them, dance and music made sex fun. Use of marijuana and alcohol helped them reduce inhibitions, as is commonly reported by many people who use them. As an important note, when it comes to how much these substances can facilitate fun, one or two drinks are most likely to make it fun, but more than that have depressing effects on our ability to engage in and enjoy several sexual acts. Finally, for Nakita and Joi, having Manny added a bit of sociable thrill fun with their typical sensual fun, but it was not something they wanted or needed all the time. They decided it would be an annual adventure, especially given that penetration was not the highlight of fun for either of them. What they most enjoyed was his companionship and willingness to be a part of their sexual play, rather than someone who wanted to assert himself as the provider of it.

As an exercise, rank these three types of fun: sensual, social, and achievement. If it helps, recall a story about a time when you've had each of these types of fun. Then, determine whether you had a chill or thrill version of that fun. Maybe you had a combination of fun experiences, like a sexual encounter (sensual) where you and your partner (social) tried to outdo each other (achievement) by providing the most pleasure. Your ranking of them will help parse out which is most meaningful to good sex for you. For example, if sensual chill fun ranks highest, your next sexual experience might include delicious food and wine. If sensual thrill fun ranks highest, you might try an exotic food or drink you've never tried before instead of something familiar. Or you might let your partner blindfold you and feed you things you cannot see. For the sexual experience after that, go to your second ranked fun and sprinkle it with a little bit of that ingredient. Repeat for your third ranked fun. The point is to integrate fun intentionally into your sexual appetite in a variety of combinations to assess which one brings you the most joy.

3

Good Sex
is Pleasurable

Steph, a white cis woman from the suburbs, had just ended her engagement to Rick. It was abrupt, but she was certain. She was too young, at twenty, to have made such a commitment.

Steph began spending more time with her best friend Sam, a transgender man. They'd grown up together and they'd been close long before Sam came out. His parents still called him Samantha, so he wanted to get far away when it was time for college. He went to school in Atlanta. Steph drove down eight hours the day she ended the engagement with Rick, collapsing at Sam's doorstep around one o'clock in the morning, knocking and sobbing. The tears were a mix of grief and relief; she'd done what she needed to do for her but knew it hurt Rick and Ashton—his son—deeply. Sam shuffled her in, warmed up some soup, and just listened until they fell asleep.

The next morning, Steph woke up early and made Sam breakfast in bed. She felt at home waking up next to Sam, like this was always where she was meant to be. They ate and talked, spent the day sitting on the balcony, then Steph's hand grazed Sam's back as they got up to go inside.

Sam felt the current of that touch travel from his back to his clitoris. He had known since age ten that Steph was one of his great loves, but he never considered pursuing anything sexual or romantic while she was with Rick. He was content with friendship and exploring pleasure and possibility with the new people he was meeting in Atlanta. The world felt so much bigger since he'd left his parents. His body felt much more like his own since he'd recognized his masculinity and expressed it more openly. He turned to Steph. "If you felt what I just felt, and you want what I want, let me know."

"Yeah, I did and do." Steph leaned in for a kiss that unearthed her, reminded her how to breathe again. It had been a while since her body felt online, responsive, craving. They fell into each other on the living room floor, kissing, caressing, making love, with Steph moaning to various types of pressure and pace with which Sam masterfully massaged her vulva, vagina, and clitoris. Steph hadn't even learned how to treat her own genitals to pleasure this good, but she was ready to learn with and for Sam. They took turns exploring ways to create new forms of pleasure for each other. None of it felt familiar except their care for each other, but it felt so good.

In our session, Steph shared, "His fingers danced inside me. Fingers, which I had come to believe were a lesser sexual organ than a penis, made magic of me. Each time he stroked my G-spot with his middle finger, I felt like I would levitate. Pleasure echoed from my vagina to parts of me that couldn't be reached with his actual fingers but were still quite touched by something else. Interestingly, there was never an orgasm. My body did not want a denouement. It wanted to ride the pleasure of those echoes, sexual sound waves retuning my frequency.

"I guess I had not been aware of how much of my sexual self was locked away during this past relationship. Sam's fingers felt like the key to reopening, and I wanted to stay open. I was open for months after that, exploring my adult sexual self on my terms. I was fumbling through it like anyone in their early twenties, and yet it felt so good."

They came to therapy together to explore how to expand their ability to offer and enjoy sexual pleasure with each other.

PENALIZING SEXUAL PLEASURE

A Google Books Ngram search of "sensual pleasure" from 1500–2019 reveals that in the corpus of all books published in English over the course of 519 years, the use of sensual pleasure didn't really pick up until around 1590, then it peaked in the 1770s. It declined quite sharply as the 1800s approached and kept that downward trend until 1917. Its use is on a slow upward trend today.

The earlier books weren't singing the praises of sensual pleasure, as you might imagine. They were often shaming people who sought any type of pleasure, with sensual or bodily pleasure being treated as one of the most shameful types. Take this 1524 text from Juan Luis Vives, *The Education of a Christian Woman*, which says, "What bodily pleasure is, how vain and foolish a thing" and goes on to emphasize how chastity is a woman's greatest virtue. Vives also states that a woman's body belongs first to her father, then to her husband, and never to herself. It's incredibly hard to achieve pleasure parity when the cultural recipes call for unseasoned sex. So we have over five hundred years of conditioning around women's pleasure to unpack in this chapter. No biggie.

Men didn't have the best messaging on pleasure either. Like fun, pleasure was perceived to be in direct contrast to the rationality and reason promoted by that era. In many of the chapters of this book, it will become clearer how the cultural mandate for "rationality" was one of the biggest barriers for many ingredients to good sex. For some time, USA society emphasized that nothing should produce pleasure, not the food you ate, the activities you participated in, or the sex you had. The fear was that succumbing to pleasure would lead to a lack of responsibility and hedonism that would tear the very fiber of American culture down. Threads of these messages are still woven through our cultures, reflected most in backlash against the free love and more open drug use of the 1970s and even against the sex positivity movement of the 2020s.

DEFINING PLEASURE AND DIFFERENTIATING ORGASM

A lot of sex research acts as if pleasure and orgasm are synonymous, overlooking the many ways to experience sexual pleasure that don't require the contraction and release of orgasm. Orgasms are fantastic for many people, no doubt about it! However, pleasure deserves to be explored on its own terms, separate from orgasms. We need to unpack what pleasure truly is and can be, especially considering the lack of "pleasure parity" in our current world. As Xanet Pailet, author of *Living an Orgasmic Life*, points out, this means pleasure isn't equally accessible to everyone, and sometimes it even gets a bad rap.

There are so many components to sexual pleasure, little nuances we may notice if we pay closer attention to what pleases us. Scientists Marlene Werner, Michèle Borgmann, and Ellen Laan out of Amsterdam and Switzerland consider sexual pleasure a state and a trait. That is, it's a state of being that comes and goes, depending on the context. Pleasure is also one's propensity to experience something as pleasurable in the first place. To take it further on the second part, it is propensities, abilities, and capabilities to experience sex as physically (and maybe even emotionally and spiritually) rewarding.

Five types of pleasure rewards, each with any number of ways to experience them, are:

- **Sensual Pleasure** (encompassing basic sensory, physiological as well as erotic rewards), such as enjoying a certain type of touch,

- **Bonding Pleasure** (encompassing nurturance, relatedness, connection, love, acceptance, communion, and attachment and parts of trust and safety), such as feeling accepted by a partner's physical closeness,

- **Interaction Pleasure** (encompassing sharing pleasure, relatedness, beneficence, and parts of morality), such as enjoyment of giving and receiving,

- **Pleasure-related Validation** (encompassing esteem and self-esteem enhancement), such as feeling desirable, and

- **Pleasure-related Mastery** (encompassing competence, agency, and parts of autonomy, predictability, control, and self-actualization), such as being appreciated for sexual prowess.

We don't need all these rewards for sex to feel pleasurable. I'd argue that if the first one isn't intact, you might be missing out, but that's just my personal recipe for pleasure. Yours may not need that variation of the pleasure ingredient. It's like the difference between liking seasoned salt v. truffle salt.

There is a growing body of research and good books on what inhibits sexual desire, or the wanting of sex, but less research focuses on what prevents us from experiencing pleasure from the sex we want. Pain is an obvious pleasure inhibitor. If something hurts in a nonconsensual way, our bodies may give us a signal that makes the behavior aversive. But there are some other barriers to experiencing sex as pleasurable that may be showing up for you too. If none of these sexual rewards have been available to you during the sexual experiences you've had to date, then it makes sense that your capacity for pleasure would be diminished. Without erotic equity, your body and mind haven't had the opportunity to learn that sex could be good. Other barriers could include your ability to recognize your body's sensations at all, difficulties with categorizing something as good in general, not enough time to experience enough arousal to make pleasure more likely, and these are just the individual level pleasure barriers. As an example, some sexual trauma survivors experience dissociation during sex where they have an out-of-body experience and numbness to most sensation. So, even if the sexual activities they are consensually participating in are skillful, their bodies may not be able to process that as pleasure without some therapeutic intervention.

Typical relationship recipes can also deprioritize more expansive sexual pleasure possibilities over achieving orgasms. This type of goal-oriented sex builds upon cultural recipes that assume sex begins at penetration and stops when someone, typically a male partner, comes. Many people are also contending with cultural recipes that suggest privileged and dominant groups' pleasure should be prioritized over the pleasure of people who are marginalized. So, for example, cis people are afforded more pleasure possibilities than trans people, where trans people are the producers of pleasure and cis people are the recipients. For Steph and Sam, this was initially the case. Sam enjoyed being able to provide pleasurable sexual experiences to Steph and had become masterful (pleasure-related mastery) in that much earlier than Steph. Sam also wanted to experience more sensual pleasure from Steph, which was a part of the reason they presented for therapy.

Other cultural recipes devaluing pleasure suggest pleasure is a waste of time that could be spent laboring. Consider the old books referenced at the beginning of this chapter. Those writers were speaking to cultural beliefs that people who enjoyed too much pleasure, or even any pleasure, were going to get so caught up in it that they would not be good workers or social contributors. Additionally, pleasure as dirty, shameful, or a religious affront may also be circling in our heads. Cultures across the globe still promote female genital mutilation under a religious banner to eradicate sexual pleasure for girls and women. To make matters more complicated, many of the cultural recipes we have been fed tell us what should be pleasurable, and in some cases the options aren't pleasurable to all or most people. Steph had been told implicitly that penetration by a penis was more pleasurable than penetration by fingers, which she believed until she experienced both options. Instead of being inherently more pleasurable, some sexual activities were promoted as the ideal by those with the power to do so. This raises questions about whose pleasure was being prioritized.

My research has found that college students held gendered perceptions of sexual pleasure. Most of the men in the study *expected* sex to be pleasurable, whereas most of the women *hoped* that it would be. Not yet published data from my Big Sex Study showed that most participants, over three hundred, reported feeling "a great deal" of pleasure-worthiness, but these beliefs don't always pan out in practice. Feeling worthy of pleasure and simultaneously being able to only hope for it in your most recent sexual encounters is the crux of intimate injustice. Everyone who wants it should have access to the type of sexual pleasure that makes sex good for them. The problem is, in many cases, people who had the privilege to define pleasure—the white cis men who historically made the unseasoned sex menu—were just making up and standardizing pleasure practices that aligned with their inflated sense of self . . . I see you Freud and 'nem.

STRATEGIES FOR SOLO AND PARTNERED PLEASURE

Pleasure can be solo or partnered, and there's a certain magic to knowing how to experience both. So, the practices that follow are going to relate to solo and partnered sexual pleasure.

The first step is to do a Yes, No, Maybe So list. It sounds so simple, until you realize you likely haven't had the time to sit and reflect on what pleases you. In this list, you create three columns on a piece of paper, with each heading at the top. In your Yes column, you write down everything that brings you sensual and sexual pleasure. Write as many things as you can think of, regardless of how others may feel about them. If you feel a twinge of shame or guilt, take a deep breath or two, and keep going. You are pleasure-worthy, so you get to—at a minimum—*write* everything down.

In your No column, you write down the things that are painful, unpleasurable, or not at all appealing to you. You could have tried them and said "never again" or never have to try them to know it isn't for you.

In your Maybe So column, you write the things that may offer you pleasure in certain contexts, but not others. For example, maybe exhibitionist sex gives you pleasure on vacation, but not in your hometown.

Once you have these written, consider them through the past sexual recipes you've learned. Are any of the activities in your Yes column pleasures you think *should* be pleasurable based on how you were raised or socialized, but not what you like? Are any of the activities in your No column pleasures you are afraid to try because of how others will shame you, but you feel curious and open to it? Are any of your Maybe So's really No's that your partner likes, but you don't? Take the time to consider each item on your list intentionally, opening the opportunity for a step toward sexual liberation. Revise your recipes as you need to.

Then, identify what type of sexual pleasure is reflected in your Yes column, using the types of pleasure list from earlier in this chapter. See what type of pleasure is most representative of your pleasure profile. For example, you may find that most of the things you like are related to bonding pleasure. This can help you be curious about other possible pleasures in that category.

Next, choose one thing from the Yes list that you can do alone and one thing you can do partnered (if you have a sex partner). If using a specific sex toy is something you enjoy alone, set aside a time for you to thoroughly enjoy it. Allow yourself not to rush, set the scene wherever you are with other things that delight your senses (good smells, sounds, etc.) and determine whether you want to devour or savor the pleasure. Savoring includes a more tantric, slow, mindful approach to letting the pleasure build up, fill you, and be thoroughly appreciated. Devouring includes a faster, consuming, delightfully chaotic approach to letting pleasure envelop and take you. Both are valid approaches to pleasure.

Whether you're a pleasure devourer or a savorer, start with the solo sexual pleasure activity. See what pleasure feels like to you. Notice where you hesitate to deepen the pleasure if there is potential to do so. Notice what thoughts arise as you experience the pleasure, if any. When you're done, consider how you knew you were finished. Next, journal about it. Capture as many details as you can about the solo sexual pleasure experience.

If you're partnered, you can try the next Yes with them. Tell them what the Yes is with as much detail as you can, including whether you want to be savored or devoured, and invite them to try it with you. You can even ask them to do the Yes, No, Maybe So activity and offer to participate in one of their Yes activities as well. If they consent, co-create the scene. Set the time and place, with enough time to enjoy the pleasure for both of you. Notice any differences in the way you experience pleasure with a partner versus alone.

Taking the same considerations above in the solo sex, discuss the questions in relation to the partnered pleasure experience. How did the discussion go? If your partner is a different gender, race, age, or ability status, etc. than you, how might that have affected the things you noticed and how you discussed them? As an example, noted above, my research found that men expect pleasure, while women hope for it. These unique orientations to pleasure can inform the way you experience and discuss pleasure with each other.

One thing to remember is that pleasure, like many other good sex ingredients, is a practice. You can't do these activities once and expect that pleasure will now and forevermore be a part of your sex life. We all contend with too many pleasure barriers (sexual and otherwise) that obstruct our ability to enjoy for enjoyment's sake. So, building your capacity to appreciate, and the skills to create, pleasure around you requires intention and time. For instance, if you choose to do just one thing, even the same thing, on your Yes list consistently once a week for six months, you may begin to feel more pleasure-worthy and able to create other pleasure possibilities in your life. Be patient and compassionate with your development of pleasure-worthiness, as you divest from all the cultural, relationship, and self-recipes that have made you feel as if you're wrong for liking something a lot. Remember, we're talking about over six hundred years of pleasure-bashing messages in our societies that you are resisting.

If you have a partner or partners, you may be in a privileged position to recruit someone else into the process with you. Having someone with whom you can practice regularly, as we saw in the fun chapter, can make pleasure even more enjoyable. But if you are solo, you don't have to negotiate the terms of your pleasure as much, so there are benefits to both.

Sam and Steph found that their friendship and the first sexual experience with each other created high pleasure expectancies for both of them, but those pleasures were specific types: sensual pleasure more for Steph and pleasure-related mastery more for Sam. In the beginning, this worked for them, but as the imbalance in receiving sensual pleasure became more prominent, they wanted to learn ways to expand their pleasure-based erotic equity. Steph never had to learn how to pleasure a trans person's body the way Sam had learned to please cis women. They assumed since sex was easy the first time, it would always be easy, and it wasn't. Together, we developed a pleasure practice for them over six months.

Steph moved out and got a place near her college, but she and Sam used virtual options to continue their pleasure practice together during the times life got too busy to travel. When they could travel, they had a habit of teaching each other new things about what they were learning in their solo sexual practices that further enriched the partnered pleasure. Steph worked on her pleasure-related mastery, finding incredible pleasure in a sense of competent sexual skill with fingers and toys. She wanted to make sure Sam was as pleased as she was, even if the activities on his Yes list differed from hers. Sam invited Steph to focus on the activities from his Yes list that prioritized sensual pleasure for him. To his delight, he benefited from her commitment to mastery. When they graduated, they moved to a little house that they call the Pleasure Palace.

4

Good Sex
is Satisfying

At fifty, Sincere was rounding out the last months of perimenopause. She was holding space for the inevitable 3:00 a.m. pajama change that followed night sweats and unexpected mood swings throughout the day. Her elders had prepared her lovingly through the transition ritual to meet them in elderhood at the end of her fiftieth year. She had the right mixture of herbs for teas and for smoking, the calming music to set her sleep ritual, and the company of her group of sisters in the community who, like her, were in transition to elder. But when they got together for their weekly support session, the topic of vaginal dryness and changes in libido were subjects that just didn't resonate. She had not had sex in over a decade, had not wanted sex longer than that. As early as Sincere could remember, she had been asexual, so although she was attuned to her yoni and its beauty, function, and changes, the one change she did not experience was related to desire. Sexual desire just wasn't her thing.

Her sex life, however, was satisfying to her. For occasional headache relief, she would masturbate to orgasm as her mother told her.

When she had been in a romantic relationship from ages thirty to thirty-five, she enjoyed the romantic closeness and didn't mind sex once a month because she liked seeing her partner experience pleasure. As someone with romantic, but not sexual, attraction, lovemaking was like cooking with her partner. It was a way for them to bond and make memories, but she didn't betray her boundaries by faking desire or orgasm if she didn't experience them. Her ex respected that reality, and when things ended, they parted amicably.

Sincere got what she needed out of sex. She was content with the amount, quality, and variety of sex she had, although it was very minimal throughout most of her life. She didn't fantasize about one day waking up to her sexual self. She didn't feel broken, as other suitors had assumed when she mentioned on date one or two that she was a romantic asexual. Dating within her Indigenous community, some men assumed she was acting white by claiming an ace identity. The ability to pass on cultural wisdom and traditions to future kids was important to many of the men. Sincere was clear that she was uninterested in parenting in a biological way.

So, in her sister circle, she shared that her libido hadn't been affected by the change. Her friends gave her high fives on escaping that particular symptom of menopause, and they moved on to the next topic.

COITALLY CONTENT

The earliest definition of the word *satisfy* literally was "to do enough." Often, this was in relation to paying debts, making amends, or meeting religious obligations, not sex. The fifteenth century iterations of the definitions for *satisfy* lent themselves more to sexual relevance: "to satiate a hunger, fulfill the desires of, or make content." When our research team analyzed hundreds of responses to develop the twenty words related to good sex, we housed satiate, fulfill, gratify, and other similar words under satisfy for this reason.

Distinguishing between the ingredients of pleasure and satisfaction in good sex is important, because they're often confused. A study by Patrícia Monteiro Pascoal and colleagues asked over seven hundred exclusively heterosexual Portuguese people how they define sexual satisfaction, and for many of them pleasure was included in their definitions, along with positive emotions like happiness and peace, feeling desired, arousal, sexual openness, and orgasm. Some of their participants also included aspects of the relationship context that made sex satisfactory, such as frequency of sex, creativity and romance, and mutuality.

In a study that was more sexually inclusive, with mostly white American cis women who identified as bisexual, lesbian, and heterosexual, Laura Holt and colleagues found significant differences between the three groups' ways of conceptualizing sexual satisfaction. For example, bisexual and lesbian women found how often they orgasm less important to sexual satisfaction than heterosexual women. Bisexual women indicated feeling accepted and comfortable with their sexuality, as well as enjoying solo sex, was more important than the other groups. On the other hand, lesbians placed a higher value on nonintercourse physical intimacy and sexual activity compared to both bisexual and heterosexual participants.

So, having a pleasurable sex life and a satisfying sex life can sound like the same thing, but they're not. Pleasure, as we learned in the previous chapter, is various forms of enjoyment one can experience in the sexual moment or not, based on their capacity to enjoy and skills to create or co-create an enjoyable sexual experience. Satisfaction can be an assessment of the sexual experience after it's done (that head was satisfying), or it can reflect the collective of experiences you've had with someone or yourself (I'm satisfied with my sex life). Satisfaction speaks more to contentment and fulfillment with the sex you're having, feeling gratified as if you got what you hoped/planned to get out of sex. It's related to the reason you set out to have sex in the first place, as well as the quality of the sexual experience based on what makes sex good for and to you.

For some, the intense but temporary joy of pleasure takes center stage in their definition of sexual satisfaction. While fleeting, the memory of that pleasure can linger for years. Satisfaction, on the other hand, offers a longer-lasting sense of contentment built from a multifaceted good sexual encounter or an overall fulfilling sex life. The key difference? Pleasure exists solely in the moment, while satisfaction allows for a more enduring positive feeling. Pleasure can lead to or be a component of satisfaction, but satisfaction doesn't have to include pleasure. This concept aligns with the experiences of asexual people like Sincere, for whom pleasure or desire might not be a crucial component of satisfaction. Contentment with intimacy or a health benefit of sex might be entirely fulfilling.

YOU'RE PROBABLY NOT A NYMPHO: SEXUAL SATISFACTION AND ADDICTION

Sexual addiction is one of those buzzwords among sexologists that frustrate some and fuel others. There is no mental health diagnosis for nymphomania or sex addiction, although there are people who hold credentials (certified sex addiction therapists) focusing on treating the symptoms people describe when they say they're sex addicts. There are conflicting theories on whether sexual addiction exists. Some scholars stake their careers on the addiction model, pointing to people who have sexual compulsions and habits that are so difficult to control that sex interferes with their ability to live fully and well. Others suggest that there is no such thing as too much sex and any compulsions related to sex are simply a matter of boredom. Sexual satisfaction is at the center of both sets of theories though.

I've had several clients seek therapy for their masturbation and porn use because they fear they are sex addicts. However, only one of them demonstrated sexual compulsion that got in the way of the ability to handle life responsibilities. Life disruption, experience of distress, and inability to respect the sexual boundaries of others, are the main criteria I use to determine whether someone's sexual behaviors are a cause for concern. People from religious backgrounds, which is common among clients I've worked with who believe they're sex addicts, often receive messages that shame them for sexual fantasies, masturbating, or viewing pornography. This confusion can be amplified by popular health websites that use fear-based language, and by religious doctrine that may directly condemn these behaviors. The Mayo Clinic has one of the better takes on this. But masturbating daily is not, in fact, sexual addiction. Watching pornography isn't either.

My team's research on messages Black men and women receive about masturbation highlighted how these messages were often negative. They came from religious teachings that call it a sin or focused on the fear of getting addicted to porn. If you feel distressed, you cannot control your behavior, and you need to do more and more to feel good, such that your life's responsibilities are compromised, then that may be cause for concern. But to be clear, everyone has unique thresholds for satisfaction, and that is okay. Even having a romantic partner who wants different amounts or different types of sex than you do doesn't mean one of you is a sex addict or a "nympho," as one of my former clients claimed to be.

People who are unable to reduce or control their compulsions related to sex are not nymphomaniacs—a pathologizing term arising in the late 1700s that male physicians assigned to women who were seen as more sexually desirous than they ought to be. From a ridiculous and outdated perspective, women experiencing symptoms once attributed to a condition called "uterine fury" (a term synonymous with hysteria) were believed to be out of control due to their reproductive organs. This presumed imbalance required drastic measures like bloodletting and torture to supposedly make the women more sexually satisfiable. In his glaringly unscientific dissertation from 1771, French doctor Jean Baptiste Louis de Thesacq de Bienville shares that he wrote it to protect young women from taking the first steps toward relinquishing their chastity. Some of the first steps that could lead to what he coined nymphomania included "eating rich food, consuming too much chocolate, dwelling on impure thoughts, reading novels, or performing 'secret pollutions' (masturbating)." So, from this theory, it makes perfect sense why I'm a sex researcher today; no one saved me from these nymph-inducing behaviors. And I don't want to be saved.

That isn't to say there are not people who have a glitch in their satisfaction system, meaning they may get enough pleasure, enough orgasms, enough fun out of the experience, but their brain doesn't process it as satisfying. The concept of physiological dependence indicates that there are natural endorphins in the brain that get depleted when someone uses a substance or engages in an amount or type of sex that is beyond their reward center's natural capacity. There are also people who organically do not have enough of the brain chemicals, neurotransmitters, they need to produce good mood states in general, so when they find a substance or a practice that can give them a shot of those chemicals, it can be difficult to stop. The chemical deficit makes it difficult to be satisfied when they finally get to experience some semblance of normalcy or goodness. In fact, physiological dependence is when the goal post for satisfaction keeps moving such that having one orgasm would have previously provided the mood boost that was needed, but now it requires more orgasms. So, for some people, their capacity for developing tolerance to good feelings and mood states is a system glitch in satisfaction.

However, many of us struggle with finding contentment with anything, and sex is just another one of the things. We are constantly consuming capitalist cultural recipes, and the marketing here in the USA is top tier. I mean, if wealthy white men want to sell dumpster fires, they have mastered developing media messaging and images to have many of us wrapped around a corner waiting in line like we're at Starbucks for mini fires for our own dumpsters. So much is sold to us, and discontent must be sowed to get us to buy it. Magazines are going to tell you that you're supposed to be having seven orgasms a day, that you should have Aquafina-level lubrication, that every time you have sex it should be perfect. Then they're going to allow advertisers to buy space to sell you the product claiming to produce those results. For ace people like Sincere, they're going to sell that she doesn't have enough sex or isn't interested in sex enough. Even mental health professionals can sometimes mistakenly diagnose asexual people with hyposexual desire disorder. This can be a problem because hyposexual desire disorder is only meant for people who experience distress due to their low sexual desire. Asexuality, on the other hand, is a valid sexual orientation where someone has little to no sexual desire or interest and doesn't find it distressing.

QUALITY OVER QUANTITY:
SEXUAL SATISFACTION SCIENCE

Frequency of sex is a criterion that usually relates more to sexual satisfaction than sexual pleasure. Some people have a certain number of times per week, or even per day, that they believe they should be having sex. Even if the sex feels good when they do get it, they're not satisfied with their sex life if the sex is less frequent than that number.

The average US adult has sex approximately once per week, but the relationship between sexual frequency and satisfaction is like a bell curve—there's a threshold where, beyond more than once per week, sex doesn't equal more satisfaction in the relationship or otherwise. Age, ability, gender, and other aspects of our identities and lives can make the preferred sexual frequency number different for each of us, but at the end of the day, the best indicator of sexual satisfaction is quality (and variety) over quantity. Other things that predict sexual satisfaction include setting the mood and good communication, something we'll discuss in a later chapter. It's important to note that although this research had quite a large sample, the respondents were overwhelmingly white (88 percent).

In a more racially representative national sample, leading sex researcher Debby Herbenick and colleagues delved into another factor influencing sexual satisfaction: duration. Their nationally representative study found men and women reported similar average durations for sexual experiences, clocking in around twenty-four minutes. Interestingly, however, men's ideal duration skewed higher at nearly thirty-three minutes compared to women's preference of twenty-seven minutes. This discrepancy could suggest shorter sexual encounters leave men feeling less satisfied, contrary to cultural recipes that suggest men prefer quickies, a la the wam-bam-thank you ma'am myth.

Many couples report that their sexual satisfaction decreases over time, even if their relationship satisfaction stays the same, but less so if relationship satisfaction increases. Something about that limerence period (the first six to eighteen months when chemicals create an intoxicating interest in a lover) sex hits different, but the reasons for sex also may change as the relationship continues. For example, the novelty of a newer sex partner with whom you get to explore may wane as you and your partner get to know each other sexually and romantically. However, for other couples this added intimacy (as noted in the intimacy chapter) improves sexual satisfaction. Again, this circles back to the reasons one is having sex in the first place.

According to Cindy Meston, a leading psychophysiological sexologist, and David Buss, there are over two hundred reasons people have sex. Some may be more facilitative to sexual satisfaction than others, but that hasn't yet been tested scientifically. After they surveyed over 1,500 people to have them determine which of the reasons were most relevant for them, they compiled these reasons to four categories: physical reasons, emotional reasons, goal attainment reasons, and insecurity reasons. So, research has shown that if you're having sex because it feels good, and the sex you end up having feels good, you're more likely to be satisfied. But sex scientists have yet to find out if someone having sex because they want to seek revenge on an ex, and the ex does indeed feel hurt by their having sex, feels satisfied.

STRATEGIES FOR STUDYING YOUR SATISFACTION

I'm hoping you've gathered by now that when I say good sex, I mean sex that is good for and good to all the people involved in the sexual experience, as defined by the people involved in the sexual experience. Satisfaction, like most components of good sex, is in the eye of the beholder.

To clarify what satisfaction means to you, chart your three most recent sexual experiences, as well as the two you'd describe as the most and least satisfying sexual experiences you can recall in your life. Consider the reasons you had sex on those occasions. What were the factors you weighed in that decision? What were your sexual motivations? For example, during your most recent sexual experience, did you have sex because you wanted emotional closeness, orgasm, revenge, to avoid feeling guilt about not having had sex in a while, to get your bills paid? Allowing yourself to admit the reasons you choose to have sex, which can be many, can help you determine your pathway to sexual satisfaction. Write them down, without self-judgment or shame.

Next, do you get your expectations and needs met when you have sex? How often, especially as there may be different expectations and needs for different seasons of yourself. If you had sex because you hoped it would help your social status climb, did you climb? If you had sex because you wanted to experience pleasure, did it feel good to you? Was the sex a fulfilled or unfulfilled expectation? Understanding that even the most satisfying sex lives are not 100 percent satisfying, because what is perfection anyway, are you able to experience contentment despite a period of low satisfaction? If it was unfulfilling, how did you reconcile that with yourself or communicate that with your partner? (One of the later chapters on communication will help you understand how to improve your sexual communication, if this is an area that would make sex good for you.)

If those sexual experiences were fulfilling, how did you express gratitude for them so that you avoid taking for granted an opportunity to have your sexual needs and expectations met? Expressing gratitude for sexual satisfaction reduces the drive to go immediately to the next opportunity or to look for reasons to criticize it. If you did not express gratitude, opt to do so as an experiment in sexual satisfaction.

Over the next sixty days, practice sexual gratitude with yourself or your partner(s) and chart how your qualitative experience of satisfaction deepens or enriches.

For a few gratitude expressions, you can say, "Thank you for meeting X need for me," "Thank you for fulfilling X desires for me," or "I appreciate that I got to share this experience with you." If you want to more directly speak to the aspect of satisfaction that made it good for you, you can say, "Thank you for fucking/making love/pleasing me in X position" or something similar. You can speak it, leave a little note, or text it to yourself or your partner. If you choose to say it during or immediately after the sexual experience, take a moment, as long as you want, to bask in the sense of gratification that comes from sexual satisfaction.

For Sincere, the gratitude, a normal part of her daily spiritual practice, also related to her sexual identity and sex life. Every day she thanks Spirit for her asexuality, such a rare way of being that has brought a lot of creative energy into her life. She thanks her closest loved ones for not asking her to be anything other than herself. She thanks Spirit that she has released the idea that she should be sexual with someone just because society expects that of a Native woman. She thanks her body during and after masturbation when it does help her headache or other pain subside. She thanks her body for transitioning into elderhood, allowing her to see the revolution of her aging, to learn what it means to be filled with hormones and depleted of them in the same soul cycle, to see that at all stages of herself she has not wanted sex, and to love this about herself. This stage in her life was another level of confirmation, especially in the face of so many scientists and therapists who assumed that she was experiencing a deficit in desire and arousal, rather than a real identity. She is grateful, satisfied in her life, without having sex. Thus, she is sexually satisfied.

5

Good Sex
is Orgasmic

Before the detour, orgasms were their playground. For ten years, Kim and Marcos's marriage thrived with amazingly orgasmic sex. Sex wasn't just frequent; it was a well-worn map that sent Kim into blissful spirals of multiple orgasms.

Then parenthood arrived, a beautiful new part of their journey that remade their life map. Like many couples, Kim and Marcos found their sex lives transformed. Kim's body, once a willing accomplice in their nightly escapades, now held the echoes of childbirth. Stimulation that once ignited fireworks now elicited a muted response. It was a confusing shift, an unexpected direction in their marital routine.

Theirs wasn't a love story on the rocks; it was a sturdy partnership navigating a detour. They were equal parents, a tag team raising their children with love and dedication. Their careers flourished, offering them individual fulfillment. They'd braced themselves for the challenges of parenthood, attending childbirth classes and reading parenting books. But they could not prepare for this.

Refusing to settle, they sought professional help. Their sex life wasn't a disaster zone, but the absence of Kim's multiple orgasms became a persistent worry. They were a team, and they'd tackle this together. Therapy became their new strategy, a map to rediscovering the good sex that had always been a cornerstone of their love.

"In the Caribbean, you get introduced to sexual things early as a man, you know? I'm Boricua, and I learned that my role was to make sure my woman was getting as much pleasure as she could from the experience. I never wanted her to feel like she was wasting her time, because I wanted to keep having sex. So I was on the internet heavy, reading blogs and watching instructional videos. Soaking up all the knowledge as a teenager. No one was gonna say they slept with me and didn't have a good time." Marcos laughed and looked at Kim with the knowing grin that she'd confirm his assessment.

"And have a good time we did." She joined in the laughter. "Marcos and I met when we were around twenty-six. Got married at twenty-eight. The first four years, I came so much that my neighbors complained to the leasing office. It was amazing, coming from a former relationship where we weren't doing such a good job of understanding each other sexually, to being invited into a sexual life where I could be taught some things. I didn't know I needed clitoral stimulation or that I am multi-orgasmic. I'd heard of the term, but I thought people were just making it up, honestly. But the more comfortable Marcos and I got in our relationship, the more I was able to allow the second and sometimes third orgasms to come."

"So how has it been for you two lately?" I asked. "It sounds like you had a beautiful beginning."

"We had kids." She sighed. "We have two now, and we love them, but it started as soon as our first arrived. Sex still felt good to me, and Marcos still had an excellent command of the clitoris, but it was like something in me had been rearranged. It took way more time to come, if I did at all. And time was something we had less of after kids. My multi-orgasmic capacity seemed to disappear totally during breastfeeding. It hasn't come back."

"It sounds incredibly frustrating. How have you both tried to make sense of it? Meaning, how would you explain why it happened?" I asked.

Marcos chimed in first. "That's why we're here, doc. We don't know what to think of it. It's been six years, and we've tried everything we could think of on our own. I'm a researcher. I'm a professor, so I made a career of it. Kim is a great learner too. We thought we'd be able to figure it out."

Kim looked pensive. "It's kind of common in my culture for married couples to stop having sex once the kids arrive. We didn't stop the sex, but it was like the orgasms were following this cultural tradition that I didn't even really grow up in. I grew up in Cali, not Japan. It's wild."

I told them, "The dope thing is both of your cultures have a rich history of sexual liberation to draw on, even if it's been somewhat blunted by colonialism in modern times. If you're willing to go on this journey together, we can draw on both to open the orgasm gates again."

"Absolutely!" they said in unison.

CLITERACY AND ORGASMS

In her book, *Becoming Cliterate*, sex psychologist Laurie Mintz describes the way patriarchy as a cultural recipe makes most people focus on penetrative sex as the main course of the sexual menu. You're not alone if you've fallen into that trap. But it prioritizes the way that only one group of people—the ones with penises—are most likely to experience orgasm. For most people with vulvas, clitoral stimulation is essential to their orgasm, regardless of their mindsets. However, what goes understudied is how other cultural recipes around who is responsible for the orgasm often place undue pressure on partners.

Our orgasms can be a shared responsibility, or a singular individual responsibility of the person who wants to orgasm, but they cannot be solely the sexual partner's responsibility. It's crucial for cis women, and other marginalized genders especially, to understand their own bodies and what brings them pleasure. Because old cultural recipes tend to be phallocentric—or penis focused—increasing their cliteracy is important. This self-knowledge empowers them to ask for what they want during partnered sex, recognizing that solo exploration can often lead to orgasm more readily. Ultimately, the ability to self-stimulate is a valuable skill that can enhance partnered sex. For some men, like Latinos and Black men, the pressure to be the orgasm producers for their partners is increased due to racist sexual stereotypes about their assumed sexual prowess. Living up to that, even as a point of pride, can be exhausting. And it can take away from their ability to better understand themselves as sexual beings.

As an example, a person can have a high IQ and a learning disability, but their learning disability may be masked because what is compromising their academic performance hasn't reduced it to a lower-than-normal level. In fact, they may remain stronger performers than peers. But when teachers, parents, or others don't realize a person is struggling, just because they're doing better than others, the person may never get to experience the peak of their potential. It's the same with orgasm and other ingredients of good sex.

The person in a sexual dyad who is assumed to be observing, rather than having, the sexual problem is often still missing out on the possibilities they have within them, because they're so focused on their partner, their partner is so focused on themselves, and no one is seeing them. But if the big goal is orgasm equity, we want to at least explore what each person is capable of. That was what Kim and Marcos explored.

THE ACME OF VENEREAL EXCITEMENT

I find old definitions of words fascinating. They reveal the original intention behind a word, highlighting how its meaning might have changed over time due to cultural recipes and evolving social norms. The 1680s definition of *orgasm* was interesting to me: "the acme of venereal excitement." More recent definitions draw upon the physiology of an orgasm, referencing arousal through "to swell, to be excited."

In the USA, orgasms are highlighted in popular movies and TV shows as easy to come by (pun intended) for everyone involved in the sexual experience. Few sex scenes depict orgasmic turn taking, which is a common approach in real-life partnered sex. Most movies prioritize the simultaneous orgasm, making it a cultural recipe most sexual partners contend with. Whether movie directors do this because they only have one to three minutes to portray a sex scene or because they want to entrench the simultaneous orgasm as ideal, the job is mostly done. Most also do not reflect the many ways one can orgasm, so we see the coital imperative front and center. Rather than clitoral stimulation, we see both people orgasming through penetration preceded by a marginal kissing and caressing session. As if.

FAKING THE FUNK: MAKING AND FAKING ORGASMS

Also important, the ability to "make" a person come is often tied to erotic ego and sexual self-esteem. While striving to satisfy your partner is admirable, focusing solely on their orgasm can backfire. This approach might put pressure on the nonorgasmic partner and leave the other partner frustrated, unsure of what truly pleases their partner or themselves. Open communication and exploring orgasmic options together, rather than relying solely on self-imposed pressure to "deliver" orgasms, is key to good sex for everyone involved. Research suggests cis women's reasons for faking orgasm are related to their attachment styles, with avoidant attachment faking to end the sexual experience faster and anxious attachment faking to boost their partner's self-esteem. The high prevalence of faking orgasms, more among cis women (over 58 percent have ever faked) than cis men, with no existing studies on people outside of the gender binary, is created by these media failures and communication avoidance. In their most recent sexual experience, less than 1 percent of men and around 7 percent of women reported faking an orgasm. In the communication chapter, this is addressed more intentionally, but it can be said here as a preview. Talking to your partner about your actual sexual preferences and experiences should not be perceived as a character attack, AND how you say things is important.

I would be remiss if I didn't at least scratch the surface of how privileging certain types of orgasm is a predominant cultural recipe most of us contend with dating back to Freud and his folk. Calling clitoral orgasms immature, compared to vaginal orgasms, especially when the people making these recipes had no vagina or clitoris, is so raggedy. It's clearly biased pseudoscience, meaning he made a theory based on no empirical evidence, but it gained so much traction because mis- and disinformation that aligns with the isms, in this case sexism, is often embraced by the masses due to confirmation bias. Basically, people typically believe what they want to believe and dismiss information, factual or not, that is not aligned with their beliefs.

A study out of Portugal by Stuart Brody and Rui Miguel Costa attempted to confirm Freud's theory by assessing the relationship between types of female orgasm and psychological defense mechanisms. I enjoy a good psychodynamic read as much as the next psychologist, but when the measures used indicate that women are more likely to have immature defenses than men to begin with, then it makes sense why we'd see results that suggest women who orgasmed through clitoral stimulation reported immature—already a loaded word—psychological defenses. Also, besides the heterosexist premise that penile penetration is necessary at all, and the height of psychological maturity at that, I would love to see this study replicated with more than ninety-four women. They lost me when they said, "Rather than being self-soothing, masturbation might be part of the maladaptive cycle." I include this study to reflect the range of sex science that makes its way to publication and informs our cultural recipes even in the current day, but studies that disconfirm the findings are shared a little later in the chapter.

ORGASMIC EQUITY

Orgasm is the contractions experienced in the genitals and pelvic floor (penis, vagina, anus)—and potentially reverberating throughout your body—that release blood flow accumulated during an arousal state, as well as chemicals called endorphins. They are registered in the brain as what makes an orgasm often feel really good. For many cis men, it's accompanied by ejaculation, although many cultures have established practices where men can orgasm without the fluid release. Less than 10 percent of cis men, compared to around 42.7 percent of cis women, are multi-orgasmic. But when we consider orgasm during the last sexual encounter, the tables turn. Heterosexual men were most likely to say they usually-always orgasmed when sexually intimate (95 percent), followed by gay men (89 percent), bisexual men (88 percent), lesbian women (86 percent), bisexual women (66 percent), and heterosexual women (65 percent). That's some unfortunate math.

Not even lesbian women are orgasming as often as heterosexual men, who out-orgasm every other gender and sexuality by too great a margin. There are tons of people talking about this orgasm gap, but the first orgasm gap (multi- v. singular orgasmic experiences) is less considered. Both are concerning, but do they balance each other out? Meaning, if one partner orgasms during almost every sexual encounter, while another orgasms during only half of the encounters, but they come twice, is that orgasmic equity?

Another consideration is that some people do not know what they really mean when they say "orgasm." Some men describe ejaculation without physical or mental pleasure as orgasm, and some do not. Kenneth Mah and Irving Binik provided a list of several ways to experience orgasms and asked over one thousand mostly heterosexual college students to select the ones that resonated most for them. Two dimensions were found: the cognitive-affective dimension and the sensory dimension. The cognitive-affective dimension includes thoughts and emotions related to orgasm, including components like pleasurable satisfaction, relaxation, emotional intimacy, and ecstasy. The sensory dimension included components like general spasms, as well as building, flooding, flushing, shooting, and throbbing sensations. They had people consider whether the orgasm was experienced solo or with a partner, and other than relaxation—an orgasm experience corresponding more with masturbation—the rest were more likely to be experienced with partners.

People experience orgasms in myriad ways. Laura Elvira Muñoz-García and colleagues studied how people experience orgasms (not just the physical stuff, but the feelings too) by asking over four thousand people about sex with partners and solo sex. The study found that overall, orgasms felt stronger during sex with a partner, women tended to report stronger orgasms than men, and straight people reported stronger orgasms than gay or bisexual people. Interestingly, the way people answered the questions didn't seem to be affected by their gender or sexual orientation when it came to solo sex. So erotic equity has incredible nuance when it comes to orgasms.

That is another reason why the ingredients of good sex like plea-sure, satisfaction, and orgasm are separate. From popular media to sex science, most people have been conflating them for decades, but they are distinct. You can have pleasure but no orgasm, as Kim had been having recently. You can have pleasure and orgasm without satisfac-tion, as Marcos had been having recently. You can have orgasm with-out pleasure or satisfaction too, as research suggests not all orgasms are positive or good, even in consensual sex. For example, some people find climaxing sooner or later than preferred is not pleasurable, and some of the contractions may be painful depending on where in the body the orgasm is experienced. Cervical orgasms are one type that may be experienced as painful. Finally, some people described emo-tional displeasure during orgasms that felt coerced or obligatory.

STRATEGIES FOR ORGASMIC OPTIONS

The capacity to experience orgasms (as many as you'd like) when desired, rather than just because you think you should, is the aim of this chapter. Like all ingredients of good sex, erotic equity to promote sexual liberation is the goal. In the case of orgasm, which has such a positive sexual reputation as the "acme," I want to avoid framing it as the goal in a hierarchy of good sex ingredients. It is, like the others, one of many ingredients to choose from.

First consider, how do you define *orgasm*? With this definition, how often do you have orgasms during sexual encounters? Does it align with the gender/sexuality data I shared, or is it more or less? Second, how does that sit with you? Do you want more orgasms, fewer orgasms, or are you content as is? Third, are you multi-orgasmic? Regardless of your answer, do you want to be?

With the answers to these questions, you can develop your orgasmic options. For example, if you're a bisexual cis man who is orgasming at the frequency of heterosexual cis women, and it doesn't sit right with you, and you've not experienced multiple orgasms, your orgasm options may include: 1) deciding how often you want to orgasm, 2) determining what types of stimulation and contexts typically occur before the orgasmic sexual experiences you've had in the past and recreating them for a set time frame to routinize them, 3) setting a time frame over which you will establish your new count (perhaps six months minimum), and 4) learning two new skills related to multi-orgasm in people with penises. Make no mistake, routine can be experienced as boring to some personalities, so pay attention to yourself during this process. No judgment at all, but see the initial timeline through even if you have to make a few changes to the practices.

This was what Kim and Marcos were invited to do. Rather than focusing on Kim's reduced ability to multi-orgasm, treating her as the problem, both partners answered the questions. I also asked them what they meant when they say orgasm, and we talked about whether they had a common definition. Marcos admitted that he was so adamant about helping Kim get back to her former multi-orgasmic state, because he'd always enjoyed living vicariously through her. We created his orgasm options plan to increase his capacity to multi-orgasm alongside Kim. They were able to set better boundaries with the kids, use sex toys together, and dig into the history of Puerto Rican and Japanese cultures to adapt some of the practices to their current life. From precolonial Puerto Rico culture, the Arawak Indigenous people regarded women as equal and as capable of enjoying pleasure as men, so reducing Marcos's sense of responsibility for Kim's orgasm in turn decreased her sense of obligation to orgasm and both of their senses of failure if she didn't. He could then focus on learning about multi-orgasm in men, giving them both something to practice. They learned about and began to incorporate prostate stimulation for him, which included pressure through his anus that helped him experience new forms of pleasure and a non-ejaculatory orgasm. Pairing that with the squeeze method, where he delayed ejaculatory orgasm by squeezing the base of his penis and edging, Marcos noticed his experience of orgasm had been less powerful prior to these practices.

From Japanese culture, Kim wanted to try kinbaku (known as shibari in Western cultures)—being tied up for erotic pleasure. For her, the helplessness due to being restrained allowed her to feel less guilty for enjoying the pleasure, especially if she knew her kids might need something. When she was tied up, Marcos would have to take care of any nonsexual house and family tasks, so the option to orgasm more than once was gradually, mentally, back on the table. She was able to release unnecessary feelings of selfishness and fear about not meeting her kids' needs and become more focused on the possibility of orgasms. Her enjoyment of both clitoral and vaginal orgasms, consecutively, enriched their sexual lives.

They both agreed the suggested six-month practice period was a good amount of time to see how things worked, and within the third month Marcos reported having two orgasms during one sexual session. He was ecstatic. "Doc, even if it never happens again, that was life-changing!"

Within a few months, Kim was back to her multi-orgasmic self during most sexual sessions, but without the pressure to perform. "Something about being tied up released me, ironically. It reminded me that I'm more than a mother and a wife, and that those responsibilities are shared equally between us. That sense of myself allowed my body to reboot to the early relationship factory settings." She laughed.

6

Good Sex
is Connected

Tim was what most people might imagine when they think of hegemonic masculinity—almost the Jeff I described in the introduction. White, tall, slim, well educated, heterosexual, cis male, and striving for a stoicism that he could barely maintain. But he presented to explore the way he was now experiencing his expression of gender.

"Well, my wife left," Tim confessed one session. I paused for a moment to observe him. He smiled as he spoke, masking the obvious pain resting in the crinkled wet rim of his eyelids. He crossed his leg at the thigh and folded his arms. I noticed his black leggings and combat boots.

"What does it feel like to say those words out loud? How are you doing in there behind what looks like a smile?"

"You got me, okay? I'm not good. I didn't think she would really leave. I didn't . . ." His voice cracked with his first layer of defense. Tears streamed down his cheeks.

After a Halloween costume party where he dressed as Julia Roberts from *Pretty Woman*, Tim realized that he experienced erotic joy when dressed in women's clothing. Shaving his legs to prepare for it, he felt connected to himself in a new way. It was an awakening of something he hadn't known was there, and, newly married, he was hopeful that his wife loved him enough to allow the exploration.

She loved him, heavy on the *him*. She let him know she wasn't attracted to him wearing women's clothes. She thought it was just a funny joke for their office party. But when she saw that he took what she perceived as an overly enthusiastic sense of pleasure in it, she asked him to stop wearing them, asked him to promise her that he wouldn't go any further. He shared that she felt embarrassed and fooled by him.

At first, he did promise. He had only done it once, and even though it was enjoyable, he didn't have to do it again. But then he began buying a belt here, a purse there—accessories at first. He had them hidden under his typical clothes in the dresser. Then he bought leggings and a skirt, which he wore to therapy. That's where we first met. Tim was my client, not the couple, so our approach was focused on him.

His wife asked him to go to therapy to see if it could help him connect with himself again. Our work affirmed that perhaps that was exactly what he was doing. Each session, there was another garment that brought him joy and a sense of who he was: gender euphoria. To be a heterosexual cis man and enjoy women's clothing was outside the bounds of his family. He didn't feel like a woman, nor did he want to be one, but he did want to be free from the conventions of masculinity that required him to wear a pantsuit, rather than a skirt, in his profession.

Eventually, Tim's wife asked him to choose. She was uncomfortable continuing their marriage if this was who he wanted to be. He expressed that he loved her so much, but he was not willing to stop this process of self-exploration when it felt like he may just be allowing himself to get started for the first time. He had hoped his earnestness would be clear to her, that maybe she would choose to stay and love him as is. She decided to leave.

DISCONNECTION CULTURAL RECIPES

Whereas intimacy is about two or more people establishing a sense of closeness, this chapter is about how you sexually connect with yourself and your body. Although gender expression awareness and sexual self-awareness are distinct, in some cases they may have areas of overlap as they did for Tim. The cultural recipes promoted by society, community, family, and especially our sexual/romantic partners can prevent some of us from getting to know our sexual selves. This disconnection, a type of dissociation, is often a consequence of intimate injustice, or internalizing the idea that embodiment and self-connection should not be available to everyone.

Around 1926, the meaning of *connect* evolved to include "getting in touch with"—often related to telephone services, but typically its definitions meant to join in relation to distinct objects or people. As an ingredient for good sex, the type of connection this chapter highlights is sexual embodiment, or the reintegration of the mind, body, and soul in a way that can be experienced mindfully. It's essentially getting in touch with yourself again, especially those parts of yourself that have been suppressed, overlooked, or compartmentalized for social acceptance and a perceived sense of safety.

Politicians, religious leaders, scientists, doctors, and other cultural recipe writers, by way of schools and even families, invest in keeping people dissociated from their bodies. It typically begins well before adulthood. Take purity culture as a major recipe. Religious leaders are influenced by what they perceive as a moral compass that points toward purity. This often means to avoid sexual experiences prior to heterosexual marriage or you're, at best, not in their god's good favor, or, at worst, going to hell. It would make sense if they preached sexual self-exploration and masturbation as a way to avoid copulating, but they mostly just find ways to use their spiritual texts to make believers feel bad about masturbating too.

Often, people who are fed this cultural recipe more directly end up dealing with incredible amounts of sexual shame when they opt to have sex outside of marriage anyway. For the people who do live up to this standard, some have lingering sexual complications based on sexual shame, even though they're married. Finally, if you identify as queer in any way, much of the religious oppression directly targets you.

Religious leaders exert significant pressure on political leaders. Their doctrines heavily influence laws about school curricula and dictate which programs and research the government funds. And since religious institutions are a large source of community for many people, even political leaders who have different, more progressive or liberal views risk ostracism from their most familiar communities if they speak out against what their religious communities want to promote. As this is being written, the United Methodist Church is experiencing thousands of disaffiliations from more anti-LGBTQ congregations who are forming the Global Methodist Church.

Bringing it to public schools, which often fail to represent the separation between church and state, currently twenty-eight states mandate their schools stress abstinence as the only developmentally appropriate sex option. These are known as abstinence-only or sexual risk avoidance sex education curricula. These typically avoid affirming masturbation, even though it can be used as a strategy to experience sexual pleasure and explore one's sexual self without engaging in partnered sex. My team's research has found that most messages people receive about masturbation are based on religious principles, such as it being evil, dishonoring God and yourself, and spilling your seed—all misreads of the story of Onanism.

These abstinence-only curricula also reject varied affirming ways of viewing gender and sexuality; they plainly prevent queer youth from benefiting from representation in the books and resources provided. Only ten states and DC require sex education curricula to be inclusive of sexually and gender marginalized people. They also rarely require boys and girls to receive the same messages, with cis boys getting the message that having sex is not preferred, but not as bad for them as it is for cis girls. Furthermore, the sex education books and materials used typically only depict white bodies that appear physically able and slim, erasing People of the Global Majority, disabled, and fat people from most sex ed all together.

Parents, having received the same or worse sex education, feel awkward or embarrassed when talking to their kids about sex. They may even feel disgust or dread when considering their kids as sexual beings, although they likely always have been and will be. Many of us buy into the cultural recipe that because kids don't have the capacity to take full responsibility for procreation, or even their own health care, they shouldn't be considering sex until they can. A part of this is also based on the capitalist assumption—that affects poor adults in similar ways as kids—that one must have financial means to be worthy of and ready for good sex. This clusterfuck of cultural recipes mires the opportunity to see sexual self-awareness through connection with the self and the body as a healthy, beautiful process across the lifespan. This is how I end up seeing grown people as clients who are just now allowed to discover something about their genders, sexualities, and selves that has been suppressed—maybe repressed—for most of their lives.

BODY AND SEXUAL AWARENESS

Body awareness is a critical component to connected sex. The research highlighting this often focuses on cis women with sexual dysfunction, but people of other genders benefit too, albeit differently. Research out of Portugal by Ana Carvalheira and colleagues revealed that among 909 sexually active people, cis men had significantly lower scores on body awareness and body dissociation than cis women. So, if men were less aware of their bodies but also less likely to dissociate than women, it might speak to our different sexual socializations.

Further, sex scientists Brooke Seal and Cindy Meston found that interventions like sensate focus, mindfulness exercises, and even science lab studies demonstrated some utility in enhancing sexual well-being for cis women. But there are fewer studies focused on cis men, and little to none focused on trans and nonbinary people reviewing the same efficacy of these sexual enrichment strategies. Men, as the standardized bodies in our culture, may not have to contend with the same level of oppressive scrutiny related to their bodies or be as aware of themselves as the norm . . . if they fit with the norm. But we know how difficult it is to fit into such a narrow window as the normative cultural recipe for most people, men included. Almost no men fit into the hegemonic masculine ideal, but the different ways they don't fit in have nuanced, albeit not any less harmful, effects.

For Tim's previous norm of showing up as a tall, educated, slender, cis white man, there were few critiques and assaults he had to navigate other than ones that came from other cis white men. As he shifted in his gender presentation, however, his body awareness grew. He used therapy to avoid turning that awareness of his body and how it was becoming increasingly stigmatized into understandable bodily dissociation. This meant he had to confront the pain that dissociation often protects people from. To do this, we couldn't just focus on the body. We had to make sure we included his mind and soul in the process.

STRATEGIES FOR BODY MIND SOUL CONNECTION

The body, mind, and soul (however you might conceptualize the soul) are connected; at least they start off that way. To compartmentalize them from each other, or from yourself, is harmful, even when it's unintentional. Even when it is temporarily protective. And the process of compartmentalization, because it is so normal in our culture, is seductive because it's easier to fit in. It's easier to numb out the pain of sexual disconnection than to engage in the work of sexual connection or reconnection. But it is possible to recover a sense of sexual connection.

Mindful masturbation can be a powerful tool for reconnecting with your sexuality. Imagine it as quality time spent with yourself, a chance for sexual self-exploration and awareness that connects your mind, body, and soul. The way you approach solo sex can reveal how disconnected you might feel. For example, if you typically rush to orgasm without much thought, consider incorporating intentional fantasies and slowing down. Even a minute extra can make a big difference. On the other hand, maybe your solo experience follows a cycle of bingeing and purging. You feel compelled to chase pleasure you've been denied, but then guilt and shame set in, leading you to abstain entirely out of fear of confirming negative messages you've internalized about your sexuality. Both these scenarios highlight the importance of mindful exploration.

MINDFUL MASTURBATION

As a change in practice, make mindful masturbation a ritual. The ritual should have a beginning, middle, and end that brings in the moment with intention; allow the moment to be experienced with the desire to integrate mind/body/soul and conclude with something that grounds you.

At a minimum, begin by saying a simple affirmation: "My body is beautiful as is, changes and all." Seduce yourself with other affirming words and begin noticing your body through a body scan. Start at your toes and touch them to see if there is any erotic energy for you. Move up your ankles and calves slowly, trying different types of pressure, texture, and touch. You can even play with temperature as a part of your ritual, by working with cool water, ice, a warm cloth, or very warm oil. (In the sensual chapter, we're going to dive deeper into this choice.) Touch the front and back of your knees, your thighs, and your hips. Allow your hands to hover over your genitalia and briefly offer them a special affirmation of gratitude. Continue to your butt, waist, chest or breasts, then shoulders. Touch each arm and finger before moving to the neck, face, and scalp.

Notice the variety of pressures preferred by different sections of your body. Notice the areas where your mind begins to wander or think thoughts that are distracting or unkind. If there are any areas where you feel negative toward a part of your body, return to that and hover over it with your hands. Specifically affirm that body part with "My X is beautiful, changes and all." The point is not to believe it the first time. The point is to choose to affirm that part of you regardless of how you feel about it. Then, return to the parts of your body where you felt the most pleasure or good sentiments, and use the same affirmation to affirm them. Go back and forth between body parts you like less and more to normalize the same language for both. Reduce the hierarchy of beauty or goodness you've created with the body parts.

Recall the parts of your body where you felt physical tenderness, discomfort, or pain. Set an intention to send healing and rejuvenation to those places as you return to your erogenous zones. Erogenous zones are the places you scanned that felt the most delightful to touch.

These could be your ears, scalp, the back of your knees, breasts, toes, wherever. Touch them while you begin to shift your thoughts toward sexual pleasure. If you can look at them, take a moment to gaze. If not, you can close your eyes and imagine what it looks like to stimulate that part of your body. In this way, you're engaging your mind and body, by way of your imagination. Your soul is the part of you setting the intention and returning to affirmation.

Finally, move to your genitals. Touch them as lightly as possible at first, noticing each component. If you have a vulva, touch both inner and outer labia, the clitoris, and inside the vagina. If you have a penis, touch your scrotum, shaft, and head of your penis. Express gratitude for their ability to create energy, erotic or otherwise. Express gratitude for your genitals' ability to create and provide pleasure and wellness. Then, change the pressure, direction of your touch, and rhythm of your touch to whatever feels best to you. The goal is not to orgasm, but you can allow yourself to if you feel inclined. If you do, try to stay in your body/mind/soul simultaneously, maintaining awareness of where the pleasure originates and where it flows, noticing how you feel emotionally, and thinking grateful thoughts for this opportunity for reintegration.

Allow the time and space to be distraction free, so being in solitude is ideal if you have that option. As you choose an end point, whether it is after several orgasms or just an ending based on the time you set aside, remember your closing ritual. This could be to reanimate—or wiggle—each part of your body. It could also be helpful to journal about the experience, while sipping a soothing warm tea or glass of wine. Either way, make sure that the capstone of the experience is just as intentional as the beginning and middle, because that allows a good container for the integration process to unfold.

Following Tim's session where he disclosed the pending separation from his wife, I invited him to do a similar ritual. We acknowledged that as he was becoming more familiar with his new gender expression, it was also reworking the way he experienced his body and sexual self. His task before our next session was to engage in a solo sexual ritual to honor his mind/body/soul as it was in this new season, as he grieved the loss of the relationship he'd spent years developing with his wife.

For him, the ritual began with candles surrounding a framed wedding photo of them, and a moment to send loving-kindness to her and the person he was when they got married. Next, he practiced mindful meditation and did a body scan, wearing a beautiful pair of lace stockings to signal his acceptance of this new phase of himself. He ended the ritual with a letter to his wife and himself. To her, he expressed that although he would grieve the loss of their relationship, if they were to end here, he wanted her to know he loved her and the time they'd shared. Learning to love himself as he evolved was just as important, but not more or less. To himself, he expressed curiosity and excitement about this new phase of growth. He saw it as a chance to explore a different kind of erotic power, one that didn't rely on the privileges he once enjoyed as a white cisgender man. He thanked his mind/body/soul for finding its way back to integration in a world that tried so hard to divorce him of himself.

7

Good Sex
is Passionate

I don't want air. I want him.

I'm barely breathing, and my body is aflame. We haven't touched each other, but we're sitting less than a yard apart at opposite corners of a twin bed with no headboard, volleying poetic verse as if we wrote the lyrics in advance. I'm good at restraint, until I'm not, so I'm beckoning him with my words to leap from his corner of the bed to mine. He doesn't move. He continues to pour poetry on me like lighter fluid. I will gladly die in this fire tonight.

I fell in love with poetry early in my life. By fourth grade, I had published in the school literary journal, but before that I used to write raps—poetry with a melody and beat. It allowed me to be creative and expressive; poetry helped me find the words to capture (or escape) a moment. It saved me in many ways. So it should not have surprised me that a freshman poet at Morehouse College could woo me with verse. I don't remember how we met, but I recall that night as one of the most passionate sexual experiences I've ever had, even though there was no penetration, genital contact, or anything more than kissing. Passion is like an all-consuming fire to which you'd willingly succumb, as Janet Jackson said, "like a moth to a flame." By the time he walked me to my car, I may have invited him to fuck me on top of it, but the passionate poetry, then caressing and kissing, were just as good as any other type of sex to me.

SUFFERING SWEETLY

Merriam-Webster's Dictionary provides an obsolete definition of *passion* that still resonates deeply for me—"suffering." In my estimation, there are two types of suffering: sweet suffering, the yearning for something you know will be worth it, and shitty suffering, like the way you feel when you're grieving a major loss. Passion falls into the first type.

More current definitions include "emotions uninformed by reason; intense feelings that overtake you; love; sexual desire; or devotion." Each of these offers one stroke in painting the picture of passion. Passion may be available in many areas of life, but the erotic energy of sexual passion comes from the combination of arousal and desire. Sexual arousal is the bodily sensations—blood flowing in the genitals leading to erection or swelling, genital lubrication, throbbing, shifts in breathing—that indicate a sexual experience may be more pleasant if it occurs then. Sexual desire is when your brain and emotions agree that you are interested in sex. You want, or feel motivated, to have sex. You can be aroused and not experience desire, and vice versa. This is called arousal discordance. But when both occur simultaneously, passion often begins.

Some historians suggest the Victorian era ushered in the cultural recipe of passionlessness/dispassionateness, especially in the sexual realm. This was especially directed toward white women. Before this, men and women were considered similarly passionate, but the consequences of enacting passions differed. As this was during a heightened period of European colonization and enslavement, passion was ascribed to people of the global majority as a social distancing move;

white men created a distasteful narrative of passion after associating Black and Brown people with passion. Because of this patriarchal/classist/racist/sexist narrative, they othered themselves out of passion all together, also creating heightened risk for white women who exuded passion. Any white women who were thought to be too passionate could be branded as witches or whores. Any poor white men who were thought to be too passionate were understandable (because patriarchy) but still a nuisance to the narrow cultural recipes whiteness created for itself. It was, however, the right of wealthy white men to exercise their passions if they were exercised discreetly so that the cultural recipes of passionlessness/dispassionateness could prevail and set expectations for everyone under their rule.

The acknowledgment or embodiment of passion, in many ways, was used to justify oppression for most people. Keith Thomas, a historian, notes that this was all to protect wealthy white men's "property rights," meaning the white women they owned through marriage and the people of the global majority they owned through enslavement and indentured servitude. This was supported by Christianity and later medicine, two major cultural recipe writers. Then, Puritans and Evangelicals in the US gave white middle- and upper-class women the option to achieve moral superiority, and sometimes even intellectual parity with white men, if they gave up their passion as a signal of their lower selves. This was not the case for people of the global majority in the Americas. Passion was ascribed to most women and men of the global majority by white people, regardless of the self- or relationship recipes they endorsed, because they didn't initially want them to have any inroads to protection or power. For example, language like "savage" was code for too passionate. If you see how adopting dispassionateness became a perceived form of protection and proximity to power, then you get how tough it can be to reclaim sexual passion once you've internalized these cultural recipes.

TYPES OF PASSION

Passion isn't something you can *choose* to feel with someone just because you think they're a good person. That prompts the question, what is it that causes passion in some instances or blocks it in others? Much of the research on passion is not about sex, but it is still quite useful in thinking about what ignites or extinguishes sexual passion. Consider sports fans. They're super passionate about their teams, right? This passion translates into actions: They buy jerseys, hats, and other team gear. They also get together to watch games and celebrate wins, maybe even throwing watch parties or attending tailgates.

Passion is a driving force. Like grit, as it relates to professional or educational goals, passion is the energy that keeps you going when something may be relatively tough. So it also serves a purpose in relationship initiation. People are more likely to experience the highest points of passion during the limerence period of a relationship.

Not all passion is created equal. Psychologist Nathan Leonhardt and colleagues categorize passion into three types:

- **Harmonious Passion:** This is the good kind! It comes from a genuine love of something and fits well with other areas of your life. Think of someone who loves painting and enjoys it as a relaxing hobby, not a stressful chore. It makes them feel good and doesn't take over their entire life.

- **Obsessive Passion:** This type starts to become a problem. It's when something takes over your thoughts and you feel you must do it, even if it disrupts other parts of your life. Maybe someone is so obsessed with their sport that they neglect their work and relationships. They might feel pressure to excel because they think it defines their worth.

- **Inhibited Passion:** This is when you want to be passionate about something, but fear or doubt holds you back. Maybe someone loves to sing but is afraid to perform in public.

Now, let's talk about sex.

Who is most likely to have optimal sexual passion (that is, high in harmonious but low in inhibited or obsessive passion)? Well, people who have secure attachment styles, no history of childhood abuse, lower levels of impulsivity or shyness, and higher overall sexual desire are more likely to experience optimal sexual passion. If this is not you, don't fret. The second half of this chapter will offer options to increase sexual passion realistically, especially given the frustrating reality that some of the reasons passion may not currently seem available to you are based on things over which you had no control, like your parents' ability to show affection and care.

I've never tried cocaine, but some research suggests passion may feel like its somatic equivalent. These chemicals are why some scholars liken passion to the feeling of addiction. Obsessive sexual passion can be intense, but it's different from a sexual compulsion, where a person feels compelled to do something and unable to stop themselves from doing it without incredible distress. Compulsion is more like a glitch in your satisfaction system—you might keep seeking sex but rarely feel truly fulfilled. Obsessive passion gives credence to the high that passion can mimic. Notably, harmonious passion is more likely to predict relationship quality than obsessive passion, so there is a balance with how much passion to direct toward your sexual relationships versus other aspects of your life that warrant passion. Passion is also related to other aspects of good sex, like sexual satisfaction—which we discussed in a previous chapter. Researchers found that obsessive v. inhibited sexual passion predicted higher sexual satisfaction when women reported the obsessive passion.

Maybe it's all these parts (the emotions coupled with sexual desire and arousal) that make sexual passion feel so delicious and motivate us the way it does. If your sexual passion is directed toward a partner and mutually felt by the partner, in some ways your bodies become north and south poles of a magnet. Unfortunately, even though over one-third of the participants in the Big Sex Study indicated passion was a key component of good sex, long-running cultural recipes block the ingredient of passion for many people.

PASSION, INTIMATE JUSTICE, AND EROTIC EQUITY

Intimate justice is all about making harmoniously passionate sex accessible for everyone who wants it. It means having the depths of your desire and arousal consensually expressible without shame. This kind of passion is balanced—it's strong but doesn't take over your life (low obsessive), and you feel comfortable expressing it (low inhibited). It also includes taking responsibility for your actions and knowing boundaries. Here's the key: intimate justice recognizes that passion can sometimes get a little out of hand. If that happens, there should be fair consequences to address the issue, not just punishment. It's easy to go back and forth between obsessive and inhibited sexual passion when the historic and current cultural recipes remain so passion deterrent, but it feels so good to succumb to it. It's like a binge and purge pattern.

If passion is one of many possible ingredients of good sex, then believing you are worthy of passion is a step toward sexual liberation. Releasing the idea that other people have the right to judge how much passion you season your sex life with is an important first step. People get to have whatever opinion they want, and due to interlocking systems of oppression, a small group of people have power backing their opinions, so you must be willing to risk some potential social rejection to open yourself to passion. Social rejection and sanctioning typically don't happen in the mindset shift, it's when you put the mindset shift into practice that your attitudes are made visible. How you talk to yourself about passion and what that means can shift with relative freedom, eventually giving you the courage to practice passion.

What would you have to risk/lose/change if you allowed yourself to feel passion, if you attended to your arousal and desire, using them as information in your sexual encounters? Take a moment to sit with that thought. Maybe your answer is your partner will think you're crazy if you're more passionate. And since we live in a society that privileges neurotypicality, meaning people with mental illness are stigmatized, the label of "crazy" holds weight. Do you want the type of partner that would stigmatize you? Erotic equity may not mean you and your partner share the same level of sexual passion, but it will mean that you are both invested in whether passion is an ingredient you both prefer and, if so, how to make sure you add it.

When was the last time you were really turned on, when your desire and arousal matched up deliciously? When you think about the conditions of that last time (who, what, where, when, why, how), consider if you felt any shame during or after. If not, you're a little closer to opening to passion. If so, talking back to that shame can help you get a little closer to the passion.

Who benefits from your passionlessness or low passion? What else (nonsexual) receives the energy of your passion? Is there room to share some of that with your sexual self, to have harmonious passion across your life?

All these questions are opportunities to determine how much the ingredient of passion is required to facilitate good sex for you.

Harmonious sexual passion invites embodiment and expression. You sense in yourself the arousal and desire, rather than being numb to it, which then awakens passion and vocalization of what your passion is asking of you and your partner(s). If your passion helps you realize you want to have sex with your person on the top of the car, you're at least going to tell them. It may not be the time and place to do it right then, but talk your shit. Because to not communicate whatever passion may be leading you could be rooted in wanting to be seen as more pure, innocent, moral, chaste, or good than you feel. Look, I'm not saying you must be an exhibitionist, but if your passion makes that invitation, are there ways you can explore that urge? What would it mean to create a less risky condition where you plan for the passion with your partner?

Twenty-one-year-old me was willing to risk it all with the Morehouse poet on top of that car that night. That is what passion ignited in me, and I said as much. My poet friend's passion was high as well, but that wasn't a risk he could consent to. So we respected that I was allowed to say what I wanted without judgment or shame, and he was allowed to decline and say, "Not now" without judgment or shame. What I learned is that poetry and passion are connected for me. As a sapiosexual, or someone who gets turned on by intelligence and creative expression, a poem could be the match that ignites my flame for the evening. I get to express that I am aroused and experiencing sexual desire. I get to articulate how I want to see that passion manifest.

STRATEGIES FOR RE/IGNITING YOUR PASSION

Passion is often one of the first things to fade in long-term relationships. Couples who have been together for years often report that they've become more like roommates or business partners, where they love and respect each other, but the sexual desire, arousal, and attraction have waned. Passion is typically seasonal, like a moon cycle or an ocean ebbing and flowing, so the first way to reignite your passion is to 1) admit where it is in the cycle and 2) normalize the cyclical nature. An older study from over thirty-eight thousand people surveyed in 2006 found that even among sexually satisfied heterosexual people, only 40 percent of cis men and 34 percent of cis women described their last sexual encounter as passionate. Only 62 percent and 61 percent of sexually satisfied men and women said their passion remained the same as in the beginning of their relationship. Men and women who reported a neutral (neither satisfied or unsatisfied) level of sexual satisfaction indicated that 14 percent and 10 percent of men and women said passion was the same as it was at the start. It's okay. Delusion isn't going to help you, so be as honest as possible about the moment you're in, as well as how high passion has ever felt for you, and how low it has ever felt for you.

Using a zero to one hundred scale, make zero the least passionate season of your life and describe how that felt. Recall everything you can about the context. Were you partnered or single? What were your living conditions? Was capitalism extracting your best energy so that you had little passion to latch onto? Were you experiencing depressive symptoms, including fatigue, sadness, and a sense of hopelessness, helplessness, or worthlessness? Was there any trauma? Were you simply raised to think of passion as beneath you or unbecoming of someone of your gender, social class, or race?

Now, make one hundred the most passionate season of your life and describe how that felt. We're making one hundred *your* most passionate moment, not what you've seen on TV or heard about, because it is important to know your passion capacity, not compare it to someone else's fantasy. Again, recall the full context surrounding this most passionate you. What was your partner status? What conditions were there? How was your mood, work, family life, stress level? Provide as many details as you can.

Last, compare the least and most passionate seasons. What things were different in those two contexts? What things were the same? After you have your range, indicate where you believe you currently fall. What is your passion profile today? It could be that you're at your most passionate, but you are ready for more now. It could be that you're closer to your lowest passion season than you want to be, and you don't want it to dip that far down again. Now that you've done an assessment of your passion profile and current position, let's engage a passionate practice.

Choose one week to chart your sexual desire and arousal. Remember these are two separate things. Anytime a thought (fleeting or full) about sex crosses your mind, meaning an awareness that you want sex, write it down with the time of day and a bit of context. If you're partnered or have a person you can trust with this information, share with them you want sex, even if you can't act on it in the moment. What you're doing is attuning to and acknowledging that desire is present in you.

Similarly, if you notice an erection, other genital swelling, lubrication, or a pleasant throbbing sensation in your genitals, notice what you thought, smelled, heard, tasted, touched, or saw. Pay attention to what arouses you, but don't rush to write about it. Savor the arousal until it passes, then write down everything you noticed. So, desire—or sexual want—can be communicated or written more immediately, if possible. However, arousal—physiological sexual excitement—should be savored until it passes. At the end of the week, what do you notice?

How easy or hard was it to be with your arousal, especially if you couldn't consummate it? Were there no instances of sexual desire or fewer than you'd hoped for? Were there more than you anticipated? If you shared this with a partner, are you and your partner in alignment on passion for sex with each other? What meaning are you making of this passion profile? Are there judgments or shame?

If so, name the original source and even the system of oppression that influenced said source. For example, if you noticed you were at work when you felt desire but didn't want to communicate it to your partner because you felt too busy, consider how your work environment and relationship to it may impact your passion. Consider how capitalism and hyperproductivity (or patriarchy, religiosity, whatever) may make you think you can't stop for one moment to send a text without sanction.

There are also some behaviors that predict passion you can incorporate into (or back into) your sex life. First, prioritize orgasms during your sexual encounters. Not to make them a goal, but to acknowledge that they are facilitators of passion, especially for cis women. Because we currently live in a sexual politic that creates an orgasm gap (see chapter 5), heterosexual and bisexual cis women are less likely to experience orgasm at last sexual encounter than heterosexual and gay cis men. Women who come often are better able to maintain passion throughout their relationships.

Receiving oral sex predicts passion in heterosexual cis men, while giving oral sex predicts passion in cis women. Notably, the inverse isn't true. Switching up the sexual activities you do—not just the same old positions and such—predicts passion, as does talking about sex with your partner (more on that in the communication chapter). Finally, setting the sexual mood during sex, making it romantic with music, candles, and other intentional accoutrement, is one of the biggest predictors of passion. Choose just one of those to begin implementing the next time you have sex and do it consistently for the next month.

These strategies are passion practices, not passion panaceas. That means everything doesn't work the same for everyone, and that's okay. What you are aiming to do is rescript your attitudes and behaviors about passion in a way that opens you to the possibility of it over time, so it does take more than a single shot of effort. Check in with yourself at the end of each month when you've committed to any of the passion practices mentioned to gauge your ability to be consistent when you can and compassionate with yourself when you cannot. Finally, don't be afraid to start again and again, because you are worthy of the passion you desire.

8

Good Sex
is Reciprocal

"So, we were in the car, listening to Lauryn Hill. Will had the nerve to turn the volume up a little extra, talking about '*to get some re-ciprocity!*' Singing all loud and in my face. I was like, 'What are you trying to say?'" Malcolm came in animated, describing the conversation he and Will had in the car on their way to our therapy session.

"And of course, I started singing louder, because, bitch, you heard me the first time," Will snickered. "He picked today to act like he can't understand context clues."

Will and Malcolm had been coming to therapy for a few months, working on how they balanced their emotional and sexual needs and different attachment styles. I enjoyed working with them because we didn't have to tiptoe or mince words. It wasn't unkind communication, just spicy and direct with a little dose of levity.

"So, what kind of reciprocity are we talking about here?" I asked.

Will chimed in easily, "Malcolm acts like he can't ever bottom. I don't even need it all the time, but occasionally, it would be nice. My birthday, Valentine's Day, damn." He fake pouted for effect, but

I wanted to stay in the earnestness of his request and understand the potential reasoning behind Malcolm's refusal.

"So, I could continue to laugh with you two, but I see that it means something that he would occasionally switch with you. I don't want to rush past that. What is the something that it means?"

"It's about balance, harmony. I'm opening myself to him, prepping for him, receiving him. I want him to understand and value what that takes. I don't mind doing it at all, but it's almost as if you can't fully appreciate it if you never do it. Does that make sense?"

"Yes, it does make sense. Malcolm, when he makes this request of you, what comes up for you?"

"First of all, it's painful," Malcolm confessed. "Second, it's just not . . . me. It isn't like I've never done it."

"Only twice . . . in your whole life. And never with me," Will interrupted.

"Okay, he's right about twice. I tried it. I didn't like it. It's on my No list, doc."

"As a gay Asian man, people expect me to deal with the pain. People expect me to be willing and receptive and soft, and that's okay most of the time, because it's who I am. But no one feels like they should offer that to me. That's another reason why it matters."

Reciprocity is one of the main ingredients to good sex, by way of erotic equity. Consent plays a crucial role in ensuring reciprocity is equitable, rather than transactional. In a reciprocal sexual encounter, both partners agree on what's okay and not okay (the Yeses and Nos). The balance of giving and receiving is also important, though the specific balance may vary depending on the couple and the specific encounter.

SHARING SEXUAL POWER
AND PLEASURES CONSENSUALLY

In the mid-1700s, the definition of *reciprocity* was "a state or condition of free interchange, mutual responsiveness." Earlier still, *reciprocal* was defined in the 1590s as "given, felt, or shown in return," then slightly evolving in the 1600s as "corresponding or answering to each other, mutually equivalent." These nascent definitions are lovely because they speak to a consensual, rather than coerced, option to give and receive. The definitions include mutuality. Whereas scholars like Sharon Lamb and colleagues differentiate reciprocity and mutuality in sexual encounters, my research team coded these words together based on the similarity in definitions and perhaps even the Lauryn Hill effect of amplifying the word *reciprocity* in Black culture.

Lamb's research suggests reciprocity is more transactional and less caring than mutuality, which they define as sexual partners sharing caring attention with each other in a way that obliges them to "see or try to know what is knowable about the person and look attentively at the other for signs of discomfort, fear, pleasure, withdrawal, or ecstasy." My definition is that reciprocity is the activation of seeing and knowing, it's the behaviors that take place once the caring attention has registered among partners. Think of mutuality as your sexual mindset, echoing Sharon Lamb's perspective—it's the overall attitude of fairness and giving in a relationship. Reciprocity is the action part of that mindset—it's the back-and-forth of pleasure during sex. Just like communication is key in any relationship, reciprocity requires clear communication about your desires. This way, you can avoid relying solely on guesswork, intuition, or perception about what your partner wants. That is the work Malcolm and Will used therapy to unpack.

Lauryn Hill's "Ex-Factor" lyrics also play well with the science on reciprocity during sex. Her beautiful vocal outcry for reciprocity reminds us that it isn't afforded equitably. Across age, gender, race, sexuality, and other identities, people on the margins continue to make similar requests or demands for reciprocal sex, because reciprocity is also about how we share power. It's a demonstration of erotic equity. Power imbalances are embedded in most of the cultural and relationship recipes we've all consumed, so intentionally addressing the way balance of giving and receiving occurs in the sexual relationship should be done by critically considering the intersecting identities of the people involved. For example, stereotypes about Asian men's sexualities portray them as sexually passive, and although Will preferred that role—his personal sexual recipe—he didn't want to be bound to it. However, stereotypes about Black men's sexualities portray them as invulnerable to pain and hypersexual, so Malcolm being able to decline an activity that hurt him was important too.

Reciprocity, mutuality, and erotic equity aren't about keeping score or trading favors in sex. It's not a "tit for tat" situation where one partner gives oral sex only if the other does the same. These concepts are all about creating a balance and harmony in the giving and receiving of sexual pleasure. This might involve different sexual acts for each partner, but the focus is on fulfilling each other's desires with care and attention.

Most studies suggest people prefer reciprocity during sex, but other scholarship suggests mutuality—another name for reciprocity—can seem patronizing. In my studies with predominantly Black people, most people like receiving pleasure from and providing pleasure for their sexual partners, and it wasn't relationship-type dependent. Meaning whether it is a situationship or a long-term committed relationship, reciprocal sex is highly valued. Black men, in particular, emphasized that pleasing their partners so that everyone enjoyed the experience was important to them. In most cases, it's a social norm to respond to receiving a positive action by offering one. However, this may not play out when one person doesn't see the other person as similar in status or worth. For example, for younger people in Ruth Lewis and Cicely Marston's study oral sex is an area where men receiving oral sex is normalized, while women receiving oral sex is special. Generational differences may exist on actual oral sex, but the attitudes of who is deserving of sexual reciprocity and who simply gives out of duty and obligation tend to be gendered, with the marginalized genders getting the short end of the stick.

GIVING GRACIOUSLY AND RECEIVING RESPECTFULLY

In a reciprocal sexual relationship, both giving and receiving pleasure should feel genuine. For receivers, feeling like their partner is just going through the motions can be a major turn-off. It's disheartening to receive a back rub (or any other act) if it feels like an obligation, not a genuine desire. Nobody wants to feel like they're receiving sexual charity.

For givers, feeling taken for granted can also be a problem. If someone feels like their partner doesn't appreciate their efforts, they might be less willing to initiate sex in the future. And willingness is important, as explained by sex therapists Lauren Fogel Mersy and Jennifer A. Vencill in their book, *Desire*. They built on the work of JoAnn Loulan, who interviewed lesbians about their sexual experiences specifically. Fogel Mersy and Vencill propose that willingness is a more important starting point for good sex than simply desire. This applies to reciprocity as well. Both partners need to be willing to give and receive for sex to be truly good.

One thing I love about Megan Thee Stallion, Cardi B, and other women rappers of this generation is their emphatic requirement for cunnilingus from sex partners. While Lauryn Hill had us begging for reciprocity in the late '90s, many women hip-hop artists in the 2020s have set oral sex as an expectation for all people involved in the sexual experience. They talk about reciprocity, being enthusiastic about giving and receiving oral sex, but not in a way that inadvertently devalues their partner's decision to give head. Some of the women rappers who call men who eat pussy "munches" play right into the narrative that real men don't sexually reciprocate, only men who can be toyed with and talked about negatively do. It discourages reciprocity, treating erotic equity in sexual relationships as an emasculation of men, rather than mutuality and respect.

This can transfer to anyone who identifies as feminine of center, such that Will's experience as a petite, Asian, more feminine presenting gay man is seen as less deserving of sexual reciprocity than the larger, non-Asian, more masculine presenting men he typically partners with. Will brought this observation into the relationship, and although Malcolm consensually tried twice in his lifetime, Will remained concerned that their sexual life didn't have the reciprocity he was looking for given Malcolm had never tried with him. If Malcolm had never tried to be the receptive partner at all, we would have considered whether some heteronormativity and ideals about what it means to be masculine were informing his willingness to even try. However, knowing how they cared for each other, and the pain Malcolm reported experiencing during the two occasions in which he was the receptive partner, it was important for the therapy to attend to his vulnerability as well. As a Black, more masculine presenting gay man, acknowledging his pain was corrective.

STRATEGIES FOR RECIPROCITY: MEETING IN THE MIDDLE

If reciprocity makes sex good for you, it may be useful to return to your Yes, No, Maybe So list. First review your Yes column and note whether the activities listed are ones that you usually have done for you, do for your partner, or if they're relatively shared. Then, indicate whether that is how you want it to be. For example, if sensual massage is on your Yes list, and you are the one always providing the massages, but you want to be receiving as often as you give them, there is a reciprocity opportunity that can be communicated with your sexual partner. Talk to your partner about how much they enjoy massages. You might find you're giving them more often than they truly desire, even if they don't complain. While massages might be high on your Yes list (things you really enjoy), they might not be as high on theirs. If that's the case, feel free to cut back on offering them and instead, ask your partner to initiate massages more often. Don't use your actions to backdoor reciprocity when you can be more direct.

Next, check out your No list. Is there something on there that your partner has shared on their Yes list? Like Will and Malcolm, it may not be that you move the No to your Maybe So column, but you can ask your partner what other activities from your Yes or Maybe So list would be an equivalent replacement. Again, the goal of reciprocal sex is not for both partners to do the exact same things with and for each other, but for each person to feel their desires are approached with mutuality.

Finally, in addition to sex acts, approaches to sex can facilitate reciprocity. Do you share the responsibility of initiating equitably? Do you both offer aftercare gestures? Whose fantasies get discussed and acted upon? These are questions to help you consider additional ways to practice reciprocity.

I asked Malcolm, "As a Black man, how have partners regarded your pain or expressions of pain? Will spoke about what people expected of him based on his stature, gender expression, and race, but you didn't speak about yours."

Malcolm disclosed that most men he dated expected him to be the top, to be strong and give dick for days. Even when he tried bottoming, his partner didn't act like he was someone who could be hurt or triggered or vulnerable in any way. Unfortunately, he was experiencing Will as telling him to "get over it" just as others had. Although he didn't report a history of sexual trauma or assault, he did acknowledge that there were a few occasions where he felt he had to perform a hypermasculine role sexually even when it didn't feel congruent with who he wanted to be that day.

Will interjected, "Well, what if being the bottom allowed you to explore that way of being, and I was gentler and deliberate with the way I approached it? I don't want to hurt you at all, so if there's any pain, I'll stop."

"No, that doesn't quite work for me still. But what if we decide that I'll more actively and readily give you head, especially in a position that feels like you're topping?" Up until they reviewed their Yes, No, Maybe So lists as described above, Malcolm hadn't noticed how imbalanced the giving and receiving of fellatio was too, so he was open to other ways to be reciprocal in their sex lives.

Will perked up. "You know, that could work for me! I hadn't even considered that, but I'm willing to see if it scratches the same itch, babe."

I added, "So, what you're proposing is interesting Malcolm because it disrupts the coital imperative. People think it just applies to heterosexual couples, but queer couples were socialized in the same heteronormativity we all were, so sometimes it shows up in our desires. Penetration isn't bad or good. There are just more ways to reciprocate sexually than penetration for penetration."

The coital imperative is a cultural recipe that suggests penetrative sex is the ideal form of sex. It coincides with the idea that both partners should orgasm together at the same time, something ostensibly only available through penetrative sex. The more masculine presenting the partner, the more they are likely to be expected to be the penetrative partner. But the way Will presented it indicated that he saw benefiting from the coital imperative from time to time as something that would help him feel understood and catered to in the way he does for others. For participants in Virginia Braun and colleagues' study, reciprocity was depicted to approach fairness, but it also positioned heterosexual men as having more agency. Men *gave* orgasms and by doing so earned the right to extract, rather than be given, one. Having been more feminine of center, in stature and in gendered expression, Will imagined he could flip the script. Malcolm, providing another lens, acknowledged wanting to facilitate his partner's pleasure and sense of power, but in a way that didn't cause himself pain.

After around a month, we checked back in to see how the uptick in fellatio was meeting Will's need of being the top in certain instances. He was loving it! In fact, they both were. Malcolm was watching videos to improve his head game, taking the whole art form seriously, which was a major sign to Will that he was preparing for him and caring about how Will experienced the sex. Malcolm enjoyed gaining another sexual skill and developing a sense of sexual competence. They both found that it became less of a birthday treat, and more a regular part of their sexual repertoire than they initially expected.

9

Good Sex
is Nasty

"I want to be dominated. I think I'm ready to try something like that," Tim said enthusiastically.

By the time we had been working together for a year, Tim had connected with himself, his sense of gender, and his sexuality enough to introduce curiosity about kink culture into our sessions. He'd found so much affirmation in sexually liberated spaces, and the idea that he would try new experiences was no longer frightening. He felt excited, and I was excited for him.

"What do you hope the experience will help you feel?" I asked.

"I'm not sure, but maybe something like what it's like to be the one who isn't calling the shots. I think I want to be freed from what people expect white men to do and be, at least for a little while."

"Oh, okay. So, the expectations you've been feeling as a white man feel too weighty sometimes."

"Sometimes. It's like, I have to win at everything, or I'm a failure, because what excuse do I have? So many people just defer to me, expect me to know things, want me to lead. I can do that just fine most of the time, but I don't *want* to do it sexually. Does that make sense?"

"Okay, I see how you're trying to make sense of this. Would you want a cis woman, cis man, or gender expansive dom?"

"Oh, good question . . . for now a cis woman."

"Got it. I gotta ask. Do you want a woman to punish you for your privilege, take it from you, but consensually?"

"Yeah, and make me do nasty things."

"Nasty in the Janet Jackson way, or nasty in the disgust way?"

"Definitely both," he said, as we laughed.

"Well, I'm excited to hear more about what you learn in this journey and how it helps you feel well."

KAMA SUTRA AND KINKY COMMUNITY

Fifty Shades of Gray certainly was not the origin of kink as a practice. Texts from Indian and Arabic cultures dating back to the Kama Sutra in AD 400 refer to some masochistic kinks like spanking for sexual arousal. However, many people still don't realize kink has a culture. Colloquial terms like *nasty*, popularized by Janet Jackson's *Control* album in 1986, reclaim kinky sex by upending the script that to do things outside of the vanilla ideal—penis-in-vagina, missionary-style sex—is disgusting or deviant. In fact, deviating from some of the common sexual relationship recipes can often help people reclaim the other discarded parts of themselves that they gave up in the hopes of belonging. Further, because most research on kink has focused on white participants, and white people have historically had more freedom to be open about their kinky desires, there's a misconception that kink is just "white people shit." This simply isn't true. Kinky sex has a long history across many cultures and ethnicities around the world, and people of all backgrounds continue to enjoy it today.

Kink includes sexual behaviors that run the gamut from BDSM (bondage, discipline, dominance, submission, sadism, and masochism) to fetishes. Popular kinks also include voyeurism—liking to see others enjoy sexual experiences—and exhibitionism—liking others to see you enjoy sexual experiences. Impact play has become more popular as well, which includes being hit with different levels of force, finding pleasure in the pain. Online spaces like FetLife.com have become havens for people seeking more information and connection around kinky experiences. Jet Setting Jasmine and her partner King Noire are master fetish trainers and have a lengthy list of potential kinks to explore and let your partner know in their Fantasy Fetish Worksheet. A few more listed there include: gags, harnessing, making home movies, and serving as furniture.

MARGINALIZING KINK

Researchers and medical professionals, particularly those who are nasty, have studied how kink has provided people with opportunities to heal, grow, belong, and get free. The Clinical Guidelines for Working with Clients Involved in Kink even exist for mental health clinicians to understand kink as a culture and a practice. The guidelines instruct providers to treat kinky clients with the care they deserve, which should go without saying. However, discrimination against various kink communities continues to exist.

The word *kinky*, related to sex, didn't make its debut in print until 1959 in a British journal called *The Encounter*. It's a relatively new word, and you can already imagine how it was defined: "sexually perverted." There's evidence of people engaging in kinky sex long before we had a word for it, as noted above. However, the term *kinky* itself is a recent invention. When it first appeared, it was used negatively to criticize people who paid for sex, particularly in reference to Wayland Young's stories. He tackled controversial themes, particularly around human sexuality, in his writing. Some of his work focused on prostitution, bringing a raw and unfiltered, but humanizing, perspective to the lives of sex workers. The audience of the day considered all use of sex work kinky, meaning perverted.

The culture of kink has moved in and out of society's margins, depending on the social climate. In times of regression, or as some refer to it—silent hypocrisy, kinky behaviors and communities experience more scrutiny, surveillance, and stigma, even though the kink behaviors persist. In times of progression, more people are willing to admit to or explore kinks that may be of interest. For example, some Enlightenment period medical texts describe physicians prescribing spanking and flogging to treat sexual dysfunction in men and women.

But the tide turned in the Victorian period, where pretending kink didn't exist and ridiculing resistant practitioners became more common. In 2023, we're in a cultural shift again toward regression. So many policies and laws are being created and passed to constrict sexuality overall, making nasty sex a less visible, but perhaps more meaningful and tight-knit community of liberation and resistance. Practitioners of kink note the liberation they experience in the kink community, and many curious people have no idea how to realize it because they're afraid to lose community elsewhere. However, there is a difference between trying out a kink and centering kink as one's identity. Both are just fine, just different levels of investment in the culture.

The negative cultural recipes related to nasty sex insist it represents a slippery slope toward deviance, sin, and harm to self and others. Often, these recipes are grounded in moral and disgust frames, meaning people actively judge and shame kinky people because they believe they are not following the will of a higher power or because the thought of it just turns their stomach. That's how the term *nasty* in the pejorative sense came to be used for kinky sex. Unfortunately, some of the people invested in these cultural recipes run major sexual socializing institutions, including religious institutions, educational systems, medicine, and politics.

Notably, these institutions also are led and worked by people who, despite putting forth policies that criminalize or pathologize anything but the sexual status quo, often participate in kinky experiences themselves. In 2023, LGBTQ book banner and conservative leader of Moms for Liberty Bridget Ziegler reported that she and her husband had a consensual sexual encounter with another woman amid an ongoing sexual battery investigation. The investigation will determine whether it was kinky sex gone wrong—without the typical boundaries established—or sexual assault. Either way, the "family values" conservatives could use the personal responsibility rhetoric they preach so much to mind their own business, rather than creating harmful policy.

NORMALIZING NASTY—THE COMMONALITY OF KINKY

To gauge their own normalcy, many people wonder how common kinky stuff really is. It's much more common than many people assume. Studies show that between four in ten to seven in ten people have kinky fantasies, and about one in five actually try it out. Here's the thing: being nasty is normal. Older cultural recipes described above painted kinky people as psychologically troubled, but new research shows that's not true. In fact, some people who experienced childhood trauma find kink helps them heal.

A study by Cory J. Cascalheira and colleagues interviewed people who used kink to deal with past trauma. People from all over the world talked to them about how kinky sex helped them feel stronger, more in control, and more connected with themselves and their partners. In their interviews, they co-created six themes: cultural context of healing, structuring the self-concept, liberation through relationship, reclaiming power, repurposing behaviors, and redefining pain. They also described the positive role of having a kink-aware mental health professional to talk through certain experiences with as a complement to the nasty sex. It's all about consent, communication, and care—things that are important in any healthy relationship, kinky or not! Some people who like being submissive (like Tim, for example) use kink to let go and feel safe. It allows them to explore different sides of themselves in a supportive environment.

Finally, research from Frédérike Labrecque and colleagues shows there are different types of people who enjoy submission. Some, like Tim, are "balancers" who hold power in their daily lives and enjoy letting go during sex. Others, mostly cis women in current studies, are "sexual subs" who simply enjoy being submissive for the pleasure of it. About 30 percent of people switch things up, so you can be both dominant and submissive depending on your mood. Professional dominatrices—or pro-dommes—are people who get paid to assert themselves over someone in a consensual, professional power share. Of their work, they described the joy of facilitating submission and being a therapeutic presence for others. So, on either side of the switch, there is the potential for good sex.

STRATEGIES FOR NASTY SEX

To approach your potential interest in nasty sex, first as an exploration, then perhaps as a practice or identity, begin with a recall of what turns you on that isn't associated with vanilla sex ideals. For example, if you enjoy rougher sex, perhaps impact play or power play may be a kink worth exploring. Or if you notice a specific body part is more likely to turn you on, spend some time exploring that potential fetish. This is also where being a good learner comes in because exploration requires inquiry. Websites like FetLife offer both information and community for the kinky inquirers, alongside people who are more vested in kinky lifestyles or identities. With over five million writings, you can certainly find out more about whatever kink turns you on.

Additionally, consider who in your current circle may already be into kink. If you're partnered and you have not had a conversation about kinks with them, this may be a good opportunity to express your interest and gauge theirs. Remember, just because you and your partner(s) don't share the same kinks doesn't mean you cannot both learn and experiment together. Finally, refine your knowledge of consent, which is foundational to good sex, in general, and safe kink, in particular. In fact, the kink community often serves as a masterclass of examples on how to engage in consent processes that are both formal and informal.

So spend a month studying one kink of your interest. Take the time to digest whatever information you find with a critical eye, while maintaining awareness of the cultural recipes you'll have to disrupt before you move forward with using this good sex ingredient. Remember that deviating from any established norms can be hard, so if you learned and had reinforced the idea that real men do not allow anyone to dominate them, take some time to journal about what you need to unlearn to enjoy that experience. Once you've done your research, plan an opportunity to try the activity out. Whether you're trying it solo or partnered, set aside debrief time afterward to check in with yourself and possibly your partner about how it was for you and them. Consider where it will now go on your Yes, No, Maybe So list. If it's a Yes, continue to learn more about it and its accompanying kink community. If it's a No or a Maybe So, you can consider trying out another kink that may fulfill some of the desires the first one didn't. Remember, there is no rush to find the perfect type of nasty.

Tim's expansiveness around gender expression through clothing was much easier than his relegation of gendered scripts about what makes a good man in disposition. He worried about being harmed, being too vulnerable, being perceived as weak to his domme, so we addressed how consent practices were established to avoid harm or repair harm, how vulnerability was a form of strength that is critical for intimacy and growth, and how all humans have moments of weakness. We assessed what value, or disvalue, he had come to place on weakness, and what it might mean to divest from that.

After two months of reading, talking, and getting to know a few dominatrices on FetLife, he selected an Asian woman who was versed in feminist domme practice and specialized in white men. Weekly, they'd meet to engage in scenes of domination and then enjoy aftercare that included an intellectual and emotional unpacking of the games they played. He felt sexually and intellectually stimulated, and she was paid well and well regarded, so it appeared to be a good fit. I noticed his mood improved and his willingness to be open in therapy increased. What surprised me most was that he said he developed the courage to call his estranged wife, after nearly one year of them not speaking. They'd never signed the papers, although for that year they'd lived separate lives.

Within weeks, she returned home, reporting a newfound intimacy with her husband. The power play dynamics, surprisingly, weren't as alienating as the overly feminine dress. It seemed like his domme had subtly shifted his overall approach to their marriage and how they did gender together. Regardless, therapy sessions continued alongside their explorations in kink, allowing them to rebuild their romantic and sexual connection. His wife even signed up for a class for beginning femme dommes. Their engagement with kink acted as a catalyst for rediscovering intimacy between them and connection with themselves, but always within the framework of open communication, negotiation, and professional guidance when needed.

10

Good Sex
is Exciting

Nakita was bored again. It wasn't an uncommon thing, and she and Joi had discussed how easy it was for her to experience boredom toward the beginning of their relationship. Joi tried to keep up for a while, because they both liked to have fun, but the amount and type of novelty and thrill Nakita needed was sometimes more than Joi had capacity for. Nakita didn't even like to eat leftovers, so a lack of sexual excitement was something she was eager to address in therapy.

"I get bored quickly with almost everything, from food to sex, and it loses its power. Even with weed, the first time I got high was amazing. By the fourth or fifth time, I was wondering why everyone else was thoroughly enjoying the high, and I was sitting there wondering if I should eat another edible."

Joi nodded in agreement. "Sometimes I don't feel like I can, or want to, keep up with Nakita's need for excitement. I'm totally fine having a meal I like once a week. She likes more variety."

"At least I want the excitement with you. I'm not bored of you, Joi, just what we've been doing sexually," Nakita emphasized, looking back and forth between Joi and I. I could see she was concerned that Joi didn't get that part, and she wanted me to back her up.

"I noticed your voice just went up an octave when you said that, Nakita. It sounds like you think Joi is judging you because of your desire for variation. Am I noticing that correctly?"

"No, I don't think she is judging me. I think she is more afraid than judging. What do you think, Joi?" It's a good sign when your client can say no and correct you, as the therapist. That let me know we'd developed a level of trust and respect for each other that was felt by them.

"Yeah, it's like I'm afraid that if I don't want to keep up, she might want to find someone else more permanently. I'm not closed off to trying new things at all, but the amount of excitement I like, and the amount Nakita likes are very different."

VALUING VARIETY AND THRILL OVER CHILL

An 1811 definition of *excitement*, interestingly, was "causing disease." It meant to agitate someone until they were ill. However, more recent definitions include "to move, stir up, or rouse." Excitement ignites the senses and emotions, whereas its opposite—inhibition—constrains them. Sexual excitement is a state of pleasurable arousal, alertness, and anticipation. But how does excitement differ from fun? As I wrote in the chapter on sexual fun, there can be chill and thrill types of fun. Excitement is evoked by the thrill type, but excitement doesn't necessarily have to be fun or even kinky, both distinct aspects of good sex. Excitement can, however, overlap with either. For example, many people associate excitement with spontaneity and surprise, but it can simply mean variety.

Variety can be a great thing, and the joy of trying new things sexually is one way to keep the sexual spice. In a nonscientific social media poll, I recently asked my community whether they preferred sexual duration (the length of a sexual experience), sexual frequency (the number of times you have sex in a specific period of time), or variety (the engagement with more sexual options). Overwhelmingly, they voted for variety. As an ingredient, variety can be, indeed, the spice of your sex life.

However, the idea that sex always has to be spontaneous or new is less about the health benefits and more about the amount of stimuli it takes for some people to feel anything at all, as well as the stressors that inhibit sexual response in our daily lives. Mixed messages about this pervade the media. Magazine articles commonly highlight five new ways to be sexually free or a new approach to the same old positions. Media often disparages consistency by calling it monotonous, but because people have different levels of tolerance for and interest in excitement and excitability, sex science could do a better job of examining what the thresholds might mean.

There are biological and physiological aspects of sexual excitement, otherwise known as arousal, as well as the cultural recipes most of us have been socialized in. For example, the idea that you must be amazing at sex as a man to be worthy of relationship, care, or recognition can plague guys before they even make their sexual debut. And if they try to take a cue from porn or other media that presents sexual spontaneity, easy arousal (excitability), and perfect performance as the expectation, the belief may be shared with their sexual partner. Awareness of what excites you and how much you need to feel excited also relate to your sexual response system.

SEXUAL RESPONSE AND EXCITEMENT

The sexual response system has two mechanisms that operate together with dual, or simultaneous, control over how humans respond to sexual stimuli: the excitatory system and inhibitory system. Emily

Nagoski, sex educator and author of *Come as You Are*, provides a great metaphor for these systems, building on the work of Rosemary Basson. If your sexual response system is a car, the excitatory system is the accelerator and the inhibitory system is the brake. Most people don't drive with both feet, one on each, such that the accelerator and brake get pressed together, but that often happens in our sex lives. That means you could be experiencing the sexual stimuli that accelerates you and have stressors or other inhibitors, like certain medicines, that slow you down at the same time. Sexual response tires just burning out and getting raggedier over time without you even knowing—that was me.

I drive a Tesla (don't judge me—it was purchased before I knew anything about Elon's politics, LOL), and it represents my current sexual response system quite well. There are two pedals, but the accelerator can function as that and the brake if I take my foot off it. It basically means I can't coast anymore at forty. I have to be deliberate about sexual excitement, because my inhibitors are just waiting for me to take my foot off the "gas."

The research points to some differences between most cis men and women in sexual excitement and inhibition. According to Erick Janssen and colleagues, there are four main reasons why men might have "brakes" on their sexual desire. Two are obvious: avoiding threats, both sexual and nonsexual (like getting hurt). The third is the body's natural cool-down period after orgasm, called the refractory period. The last one is stress—too much of it can put a damper on things. How much excitement and inhibition you have might be a mix of your genes and your experiences, but the key takeaway is this: too much inhibition can lead to trouble getting excited, while too little can make you take unnecessary risks. For the men, there were three key factors: excitement, fear of messing up in bed (performance failure), and worrying about things like STIs or unplanned pregnancies (performance consequences). Excitement stands alone, meaning there were no subcategories to it. And the other two factors are subcategories under inhibition. Interestingly, masturbation was linked more to excitement than partnered sex. But that makes sense, because when you're flying solo, there's less pressure to perform perfectly.

Researcher Deanna Carpenter and colleagues took it further by comparing how cis men and women experience sexual excitement and inhibition, and some interesting things emerged. Women were more likely to be affected by mood than men. Feeling angry with a partner? Not exactly a mood setter for most women. Reading erotic stories helped some women feel more aroused, but this wasn't as significant for men. Overall, women in the study reported feeling less aroused and more easily turned off than men. Disconnecting emotionally from their partner seemed like a bigger turn-off for women compared to men. It's important to remember this study focused on younger participants. Just like your favorite jeans might not fit the same way over time, our sexual excitement options can change as we age, learn more about ourselves, and have more experiences. Scientists are still figuring out how these differences change as we get older, but therapists have some insights.

For someone like Nakita, it may seem like she had more gas and fewer brakes than Joi. She was willing to take more risks and introduce more variety to their sex life, but she also reported boredom with sex acts that used to be exciting if they did them too much. Research frames this as subjective sexual arousal, since it is based on what she says, rather than how her genitalia are responding. Put differently, she could feel bored with sex that still gets her physically aroused. That's called arousal non-concordance—the gap between experiencing genital arousal (blood flow, engorgement, lubrication, and other physiological sexual responses) and feeling turned on mentally and emotionally. Something in her brake system may have been quickly

activated with too much sexual sameness, but the brakes may not have
been affecting her body.

STRATEGIES FOR SEXUAL EXCITEMENT:
TURNING YOURSELF ON AND OFF

How many sex acts or positions have you tried? When you happen
upon a good one and it becomes a favorite, are you more likely to stick
with that one or keep trying new things? That may help you discover
your need for sexual excitement. If you're like Nakita, even finding
a really good position doesn't mean it is the one you do all the time.
To her, there is possibly another position out there that could be just
as good or better, so you have to keep the variety coming to happen
upon it. Her sexual excitation draws from novelty. Boredom is her
brake pedal.

For Joi, once she finds a good position, she wants to incorporate
it regularly. It doesn't mean she doesn't mind continuing with variety,
but having something she knows is reliably good that she can return
to helps her feel grounded, rather than listless. The reliability of the
pleasure she'll experience with that position allows her to accelerate
sexually. The overwhelm from having too many options, with no sense
of whether they'll be enjoyable, is one of her brakes.

Then there are people in the middle, depending on what it is.
Regardless, there's nothing wrong with any of these ways of being.
We each tolerate the experience and desire for excitement differently.
Esther Perel developed a simple exercise to help you better understand
your eroticism and arousal. Similar to the Yes, No, Maybe So list you
may have completed earlier, this one asks you to list two columns: "I
turn myself on when . . ." and "I turn myself off when . . ."

Using this language helps each person own their part in the sexual
excitement and inhibition they experience, rather than putting the

onus on their partner. To the extent that at least some sexual response is guided by choice, this list helps with the parts that can be changed, if desired. The first column of the list are your sexual accelerators, and different from what is on your Yes list, these are usually nonsexual or presexual experiences that prepare you for good sex. For example, "I turn myself on when I learn about a new sexual position to try with my partner." The second column of the list are your sexual brakes, and different from your No list, which are sexual activities you'd prefer not to engage in, this is what contexts contribute to less arousal. For example, "I turn myself off when I am unable to engage my favorite sexual activity."

These are all sexually subjective. Remember earlier we discussed that your mind and emotions may turn off, even if your genitals don't, and vice versa. Also, turn-ons and turn-offs are neither good nor bad. This exercise helps you better understand yourself. It also helps you communicate with your partner, what brakes and accelerators are activating during your sexual experiences, especially if your body is communicating arousal that you don't feel.

Once Nakita and Joi wrote their lists, they weren't surprised to see differences in the turn-ons, but the turn-offs were mostly the same. Nakita just had more turn-ons than Joi, and Joi had more turn-offs. So Nakita was tasked with focusing a bit more of her attention on reducing their turn-offs, which in turn allowed Joi to focus more on exploring each of the turn-ons. Each month, Nakita took care of one turn-off, starting with a shared one of making sure anything that angered or frustrated one of them didn't linger. They brought those topics into therapy more readily so we could use that time and prevent them from taking too much time with it at home. Joi went down the list of shared turn-ons first, taking one a month as well. By month six, when she got to the turn-ons that were on Nakita's list but not hers, the sex was so good she didn't feel as anxious about trying a new thing or helping Nakita try it on her own. For example, one of Nakita's turn-ons was dancing, so she gifted her a dance class package for the month. Even though Joi didn't attend, she got to benefit from Nakita's sexual excitement on Thursday evenings. The consistency of knowing "Throw it back, Thursdays" was on their schedule was even more of a turn-on for Joi, because she could look forward to something consistent to set her brakes at ease.

11

Good Sex
is Loving

The love Steph and Sam had for each other was old, pre-dating their sexual debuts or even puberty. They were kids when they met, and platonic, youthful love came easy and without pretense. Their early pictures included toddler tap classes with their arms wrapped around each other, both in pink bows and leotards. By middle school, as Sam was transitioning, the grunge phase allowed him to survive as not quite out to his parents via tomboyhood, but Steph knew. She was the first one he told he was trans, because he knew she'd love him still. However, once Steph and Sam decided to join lives and be romantically and sexually partnered, loving soon had different cultural recipes attached to it. The way platonic love, romantic love, and sexual love are portrayed as differentially valuable hit home. They struggled with the wax and wane of love as an emotional state and how that impacted their sex life together.

"Coming into myself as a trans man, I think I initially picked up on some weird, toxic masculinity stuff that got in the way of me simply loving women. I wanted to belong to the boy's club. Our middle and high schools didn't have many out kids, so I felt like I had to pick.

Guys had really different ways of expressing and showing love. For a while, Steph was my only real friend. We loved each other no matter what," Sam shared.

"Yeah, he definitely went through an asshole phase, trying to be a typical high school boy rather than himself." Steph laughed. "But of course I loved him, and I still do. It just feels like there are pressures to loving now that we are romantically committed. Friendship is cool. I have that with a lot of people though. Sexually, we're feeling limited by what love means for us. It feels like there is a certain way sex should be for people who love each other."

TO CHERISH AND DELIGHT IN

Early definitions of *love* included "to cherish or delight in." Love as action is foundational to how bell hooks explains the function of love. What is most central to her book *All About Love* is that love is often theorized and less often practiced, meaning many scholars and people talk a good game and are able to articulate what love should be, but when it comes down to acting in a loving manner, most people struggle to treat people we say we love with "care, commitment, knowledge, responsibility, respect, and trust." Being loving can be a seasoning of good sex, but it's important to note that being loving isn't the exclusive disposition of people in committed relationships. The commit hooks describes isn't about monogamy. That's where many people get the game fucked up. Being loving is about acting as if any person you have sex with, even casual partners or one-night stand partners, deserve to be treated with respect and care, and shown love through action. Even the sexual acts of love are often relegated to the slow, sensual, looking eye-to-eye lovemaking. But doggy style and kinky sex can be loving too. Love is in the approach and intention to these sex acts.

The idea of love has been warped by some interpretations of Puritan beliefs. These views make it seem like love is only for one person, or a very limited type of relationship. This misuse of love is built on a shaky foundation, just like many of the outdated cultural recipes we learn about love. The truth is, everyone deserves love, and it can come in many forms.

LOVE AND INTIMATE JUSTICE

Sometimes, after a sexual encounter, we just want to retreat and avoid connection. As discussed in the chapter on intimacy, maybe the fear is that closeness with another person will be overwhelming, or maybe we worry it won't be enough. But what if love, in a sexual context, could be something simpler? Love can be about basic human kindness. Honesty, communication, respect, and care are all gifts you can give to yourself and your partner, regardless of your long-term plans. Setting boundaries about how you want to be treated lets your partner know you value a kind and respectful dynamic, even in casual encounters. This can pave the way for loving sexual experiences that go beyond just the physical. As bell hooks notes, there can be no love without justice. Love is, in fact, central to intimate justice.

There are, like most aspects of good sex, barriers that get in the way of it being loving. Cultural recipes about who deserves love, what love means, which types of love are legitimate, and the way they interact with oppression are front and center. Sexism and patriarchy, for example, would have some men believe that if they are loving toward a hookup partner, they are weak, lower status beta men. These distasteful cultural recipes actively disincentivize men from cultivating the skills of love.

Also, consider a more specific example of sex workers, including everyone from OnlyFans entertainers to strippers. People who make their livelihood engaging in sexual acts are often disregarded, disrespected, and shamed for their profession, despite it being quite a popular industry. People pay for sex every day, and I want to imagine a world where the patron doesn't perpetuate disgust or disdain toward a sex worker following their encounter. The reason sex workers can be easily killed by serial killers is because it's commonly known that most people think they're disposable. Being sexually loving is regarding all humans, all sex partners more specifically, as worthy of love.

The exploration of withholding love and its impact on intimacy can benefit from a historical perspective, particularly regarding relationships between white men and Black women in the southern United States. Laws like those against miscegenation (marriage between races) created a strange paradox. While marriage was illegal, sex wasn't. Rape wasn't illegal either. This led to a situation where white men could express physical desire for Black women but not romantic love, a clear example of how love and sex were seen as separate entities.

The resulting systems of racial oppression further complicated matters. The "quadroon" and "octoroon" classifications arose from these relationships, highlighting the hypocrisy of denying Black women love while exploiting them sexually. High-end brothels in New Orleans, for instance, offered Black women of mixed race as a "premium" service, demonstrating a market for their beauty yet denying them the love afforded to white women.

While most Black women wouldn't have desired marriage to their white exploiters and rapists, these legal codes solidified a hierarchy of who deserved love. Monogamous, married love became the ideal, and those outside this structure, like Black women in this context, were deemed unworthy. That isn't to say that all sexual and romantic love should end in marriage, but current and historical social structures celebrated marriage as an ideal sexual relationship structure, while denying Black people access. This historical example underscores the complex relationship between love and sex, and how gendered racist power dynamics can distort their natural connection.

In contrast, for men who may have wanted to love, have sex with, and marry other men, both the sex acts and the marriage option were banned up until 2003 when the Supreme Court banned sodomy laws. The laws came with colonizing white people from England, and they were written into most state laws as each was founded. Many nations globally are still in a cycle of writing and resisting sodomy laws. Notably, sodomy, at some historical moments, has included any non-procreative sexual activities, from masturbation to anal sex. The idea that none of these sex acts could be loving has been the foundation of many cultural recipes.

LOVING SEX AS A CORRECTIVE

People often assume that loving sex is different in tempo and sensuality than other forms of sex. We refer to it as making love and offer it as a contrast to fucking someone, which is supposedly more aggressive, less emotional, and more about the outcome of pleasure and orgasm than other reasons people engage in sex. This isn't the case. The kinkiest, most consensually nasty, aggressive sex can be loving. The most vanilla bean, plain, passive sex can be unloving. Some of us have been socialized not to know the difference, because the world has been so actively insistent on withholding love from us. And the more marginalized identities you have, the more the current cultural recipes try to treat you as unworthy of love. Poor, unlovable. Not stereotypically attractive, unlovable. Fat, unlovable. Old, unlovable. Loving sex is a corrective for this.

What we seek to share or give in a sexual experience is what makes it loving or unloving. Aftercare is one of many examples. Once you and your partner consider the sexual experience to be over, how do you offer each other care? What do you do with and for each other to show love? Are you quick to walk them to the door without many words? Are you interested in talking or making them tea, getting a warm towel, washing their back in the shower? Can you differentiate being loving—showing a sexual partner love—from wanting to pursue commitment, if that isn't what you desire?

The last question is where many people who may have good intentions struggle. They don't want to lead sexual partners on by showing them love because they are aware they're not interested in long-term commitment. Honest communication is key, but it can't completely shield someone from disappointment if they crave a deeper connection. Their disappointment is not your responsibility, especially if it comes at the sacrifice of your boundaries.

I once dated someone with whom I wanted a romantic commitment, and I was aware that if we weren't moving in that direction, it might not be a good idea for me to have sexual intercourse with him. I wanted to, and I felt physically turned on by him during our make out sessions. But his careful, yet direct and honest, communication with me allowed me to hold the boundary I needed, just as he held his. We were able to stop dating respectfully, knowing neither of us betrayed ourselves in the hope that feelings would change.

In committed relationships, unspoken expectations about love can lead to inauthentic behavior. Instead of communicating our preferences for how we prefer love be expressed ("love languages" have been refuted scientifically, even though they are meaningful categories for many people), we often try to fulfill what we think our partner needs. This assumption that partners should "just know" is flawed. Learning new ways of expressing love takes time and effort, especially in a society that often downplays the importance of healthy love expression. Both awareness and practice are crucial. You can directly tell your partner about specific actions that demonstrate love for you, whether it's in the bedroom or elsewhere in the relationship. However, if these actions aren't already part of their repertoire—even if they tried them during the initial "honeymoon" phase—it may take repeated communication to get what you desire. Changing relationship habits can be a slow process, requiring effort and intention. Some experts suggest it can take over a year. The question then becomes: are you patient enough for this process? No shame or blame, either way.

TYPES OF LOVE

What Steph and Sam, like many couples, were contending with was the distinction between passionate and companionate love. Elaine Hatfield and Richard Rapson provided an overview of how these different types of love related to good sex and some of the other components that make it up that have been discussed in this book. Passionate love—or being in love—was something that they desired in the context of their romantic relationship. Companionate love— loving each other—was something they had already cultivated over time. The former is closer to the sexual arousal brain circuitry than the latter, which is why it feels so good and why Steph and Sam craved it. However, passionate love also shuts down critical thinking brain capacity while it turns up rewards. Because this couple had known each other for years as friends already, they were fully capable of the critical thinking part with each other . . . even if they didn't quite want to be.

Robert Sternberg's triangular theory of love breaks the types of love down even further, based on the combination of three components that people can feel within a relationship dynamic: passion, intimacy, and commitment. Defined slightly differently than this book, their version of passion is sexual and romantic feelings brought on by physical attraction. He agrees, however, that passion is a motivational force experienced early in romantic relationships, which most people can't decide to feel or control. Their definition of intimacy is like the one in this book: various forms of closeness with another that create familiarity and warmth. Commitment is defined as a decision to maintain the relationship to the best of their ability. Commitment acknowledges love as a choice. Various combinations of these three factors create seven types of love:

- Romantic love is composed of passion and intimacy.

- Infatuation is passion.

- Companionate love is composed of intimacy and commitment.

- Liking (also known as friendship) is intimacy.

- Fatuous love is composed of passion and commitment.

- Empty love is commitment.

- Consummate love is the highest form of love, according to Sternberg, and it includes an equal portion of passion, intimacy, and commitment.

What is important about the commitment component is to not allow it to be laden with mono-normative assumptions that real love requires long-term romantic exclusivity, and it must be between only two people. Although commitment and monogamy are relationship options that work for many people, they are not the only ways of loving. USA divorce rates also show that they don't work for around half of people in many ways.

Sam and Steph were firmly in companionate love with an initial dash of consummate love that they deeply desired to return to. So, in addition to the exercises to increase passion so they could revisit and sustain the consummate love they were hoping for, we were able to build upon their existing intimacy and commitment. This complemented previous work we'd done to ensure their sex life was pleasurable, as they redefined what loving sex could be for them.

STRATEGIES FOR AFFIRMATION, CARE, AND HONESTY AS LOVING SEX

Take a moment to explore your own beliefs—your self recipes—about love. Consider how media, family dynamics, religious teachings, your friends' experiences, and even past relationships have shaped your understanding. What messages did you receive about love growing up? Do you crave the passionate intensity of romantic love, the deep connection of companionate love, or perhaps something else entirely? After journaling about your love beliefs, review the seven types of love and select the one you prefer to experience and express at this moment in your life, while remaining open to the reality that the type of love you want may change. Which aspects of love—passion, intimacy, commitment—does your type of love need? Determine if you and your sexual partner both have the capacity for the type of love you desire. If not, communicate honestly. For example, if you want consummate love, but you need to work on your trust issues before you can commit, tell your sexual partner the truth.

Regardless of the type or length of relationship you desire, affirming the inherent worth of yourself and your partner is a core principle of love. This means recognizing that their value and yours are not conditional on the relationship itself, whether it's a casual encounter, a committed marriage, a throuple, or something in between. As bell hooks emphasizes, self-love is a cornerstone of loving others. While the popular myth that you must love yourself *before* you love others isn't accurate, loving yourself is still essential. We learn to love ourselves in relationship with others, and you need to participate in that process actively.

One way to affirm your sexual partner is noticing and naming their inner and outer beauty. This can be done before, during, or after sex. If you appreciate the beauty of your partner's fupa (fatty upper pubic area), say so. Also, kiss it and touch it like you love it. If your partner loves your beautiful way of thinking, wouldn't it be loving if they shared it with you? Affirmation is a free way to express love, but make sure it is honest based on how you really feel. Inauthentic affirmation falls flat.

Sam and Steph's exploration of loving sex revealed differences in their expectations for love within different relationships. Sam valued body affirmation during sex, especially from Steph, who knew him both before and after his transition. He didn't want to feel like a fetish or an object, and Steph navigated this by expressing her attraction, including his scars, but avoiding comments solely focused on the physical changes. For arousing love during more intense sex, they discovered "praise kinks," where verbal expressions of enjoyment became part of their loving sexual dynamic. Importantly, they both valued physical intimacy equally, and verbal praise for their mutual pleasure became a key component of their loving sex.

As discussed earlier, showing care for your partner is another facet of love. Unfortunately, traditional gender roles can influence how care is expressed. Sam and Steph recognized that their aftercare routine had become unintentionally gendered. Rekindling their romance highlighted Sam's internalized ideas of masculinity, leading him to rely on stereotypical expectations of male behavior rather than his own authentic expression. While still committed to Steph's pleasure, his initial approach to aftercare felt restricted by these expectations. To address this, they adopted a more balanced approach: taking turns being the "big spoon," offering to clean each other up, and using warm towels—all small gestures that showed care without relying on gendered roles. Similarly, they alternated initiating romance and sex, opening doors, and paying for meals—all expressions of care that went beyond the bedroom.

Being honest with each other that they were not feeling the type of love they desired was scary for both of them, but sharing it opened up an opportunity for them to work toward consummate love once again.

12

Good Sex is Spiritual

Sincere was hoping to explore the spiritual possibilities of sex in therapy. Although pleasure and desire were not her motivators, gaining insight into how sex could be a source of connection to the divine piqued her curiosity. She had happened upon a video that discussed decolonizing sexuality when looking for resources about being asexual. And moving into her elder role, she felt more eager to provide wisdom to the next generation. She had a feeling spiritual sex would be relevant.

"My tribe is still feeling the consequences of colonization on our sexual lives. I feel like I have a particularly close read on it as an asexual woman, because there used to be a sacred spiritual place for someone like me, central to our Indigenous ways."

"I'd love to hear more about how it reached you. What happened there?" I asked.

"When my parents went to boarding school and got brainwashed, they brought those white religious teachings home," Sincere explained with frustration. "They did try to balance it with some of our history though. What it made for was a complicated life of being not sexual up until a certain age—easy for me—then being expected to suddenly be romantically and sexually ready and available for a good Christian Indian man who could impregnate me and take care of our little family. The idea that I might be a lesbian was offensive to the nation, not just my family. They couldn't even conceive of an asexual me. They had long forgotten that being asexual used to be reflected as closest to our ancestors, not on the margin or out of favor with it," said Sincere.

"Yes to reclaiming your heritage in a way that works for you. We can explore some of the ways spirituality can be detached from the colonial vantage point. There is much to explore there, whether you're having sex or not."

MORE THAN RELIGIOSITY

Tracing the way *spiritual* has been defined over time, I find this early definition from the twelfth century beautifully captures it as "of or pertaining to breath, breathing, wind, or air." Over time, the definition expanded to encompass the soul and religious matters. This shift can lead to confusion between spiritual and religious, but there's a key difference. Think of spirituality as a broad umbrella. Religion is one way to express spirituality, but not the only way. Some argue that focusing solely on religious rituals can actually distance you from a more personal spiritual connection with the divine, while others argue that the structure of religion is a necessary hedge to keep them disciplined and safe.

Both spiritual and religious paths often use rituals to connect with something beyond ourselves, whether it's God, a higher power, nature, or a sense of something greater than the physical world. Making sense of the meaning of life or giving greater purpose to life are other uses of spirituality. However, religions tend to have more established rules and doctrines. Religious rules define what rituals, values, and beliefs are considered "correct" within that tradition. For example, Abrahamic religions (Christianity, Islam, Judaism) have sacred texts that outline their core values. However, scholars point out that these texts can be interpreted in different ways, sometimes leading to seemingly contradictory ideas within the same scripture. Additionally, translations and revisions over time can add to the complexity. The organizations who do the translations subtly embed values in their interpretation. Finally, consider the influence of social and political forces. Throughout history, religious leaders have sometimes used their positions to justify oppression based on colonialism, patriarchy, racism, or economic systems. This can lead to a disconnect between the core spiritual message and the way some religious institutions operate. The history of sexual abuse scandals throughout the Catholic Church serve as an example.

So, with this background, it is easy to see how experiencing sex as spiritual, when religious leaders misrepresent it as otherwise at best or antithetical at worst, can be difficult for many people. For people who have experienced religious marginalization—basically anyone who isn't Christian in the USA—conceiving of spirituality in sex may feel like a betrayal. Also, for queer people who have been excommunicated from religious communities due to oppression of their sexual and/or gender identities, associating sex and spirituality can feel downright disrespectful.

SEX-NEGATIVE RELIGIOUS RECIPES

Religious sexual recipe writers are some of the most prominent voices in sex negativity. People use them to limit what sex can be because control often feels less risky than care. Control is much less vulnerable. Religious leaders can mask it as discipline, obedience, or morality, but the tendency to ostracize any person or community from their rightful place as a divine being worthy of all things sacred due to any aspect of their identity comes from a place of control and disgust. Shaming is a primary tactic used by people who operate through control, disgust, and fear. Erasure is another tactic, such that we see books being banned that uplift queer communities by people and agencies invoking religious texts and values. As referenced in another chapter, Moms for Liberty co-founder Bridget Ziegler and her husband, Christian, could have just quietly enjoyed a threesome and consensual voyeurism instead of minding other families' business, but now they're wrapped up in a scandal that stands in contrast to the anti-LGBTQ book banning campaign and sexual rights in general. Maybe they wouldn't have allegedly committed the third-degree felony of video voyeurism had they been less constricted by the impression management of pretending to support Christian values and parents' rights, rather than control of other people.

For many people who see sexual liberation as an important direction for cultural recipes to move, the frustration isn't even that some people hold religious values that may lean conservative. It's that they take it upon themselves to coalition build and impose those values on everyone else. It's also that they think living by those values makes you a better person than others, worthier of all the good life has to offer, higher on the human hierarchy. Rather than letting whatever god they serve decide that, they attempt to make it so on Earth right now.

But spiritual practices do not have to be associated with any religion. In fact, many societies precolonization included sexual acts as components of their spiritual practices because they felt certain sexual experiences brought you closer to realizing the divinity in yourself and others. Mutual masturbation is one example. Some Indigenous tribes, especially among people who were also genderfluid and expansive, used mutual masturbation as a community building activity with a spiritual undertone. When European colonizers observed this behavior, they took strides to eradicate it based on their sense of disgust and misunderstanding. Additionally, orishas from Yoruba spiritual traditions include sexuality as a featured strength among Oshun. Zelaika Hepworth Clarke, a decolonial eroticologist, has offered a groundbreaking perspective on Osunality in sexology. Her process for auto-sexual decolonization ends with recognition of spiritualities.

SPIRITUAL SCIENCE

The spirituality framework developed by Marina Aline de Brito Sena and colleagues provides a research-based way to conceptualize spirituality and health that has implications for good sex. This framework has three nonhierarchical, dynamic axes. The first axis is the spirituality starter point—beliefs, practices, and experiences that promote connection to the second axis. This second axis consists of eight options that may work individually or in concert:

- **Sacred:** Think of sacred things as extraordinary, beyond everyday life. They could be objects, symbols, or places that spark a deep sense of meaning or connection for an individual or their religious/spiritual group. Imagine a stunning sunset or a family heirloom that makes you feel a powerful connection to something bigger than yourself.

- **Life After Death:** This refers to the belief that some part of us, like the soul or spirit, lives on after the body dies. This idea is found in many religions like Catholicism, Judaism, Hinduism, and Buddhism.

- **Spiritual Beings:** These are nonphysical beings like spirits, ghosts, or even ancestors who are believed to be able to interact with the physical world. Some people may experience these connections through feelings or unusual events.

- **Divine, God:** This refers to believing in one or more powerful deities often associated with the heavens. It's a core concept in many religions.

- **Self:** Spirituality is also about connecting with yourself, your body, and your inner strength.

- **Community:** Feeling a deep connection with others, like your family, neighbors, or a spiritual group, is an important part of spirituality for many people.

- **Nature:** Some cultures view nature as a sacred expression of something greater. This is called ecospirituality and is found in traditions like Aboriginal cultures and Celtic religions.

- **Art:** Creating or experiencing art like music, dance, or visual arts can be a deeply spiritual experience. It can evoke awe and a sense of connection to something beyond ourselves. Think of beautiful music that moves you or a spiritual dance ritual.

The third axis includes "development of values, personal growth, and sensations of meaning, purpose in life, well-being, support, and inner peace through connection with something that can affect the behavior of the individual." Taken together, these are the components of spirituality that serve as an ingredient to good sex. For instance, feeling connected to something sacred (like a deep love or a sense of awe) might lead you to use sex to strengthen that connection with your partner. Additionally, understanding the divinity of nature might inspire someone to explore ecosexuality—or the concept of nature as a sensual or romantic space.

In contrast, religiosity is often associated with sexual shame, but it also reduces some forms of sexual risk. For example, religious young people make their sexual debut later and have fewer partners than their nonreligious peers, but they do not differ on condom use once sexually active. Sexual sanctification, or seeing sex as a sacred act, serves as a buffer against sexual shame negatively impacting sexual satisfaction. All groups, particularly those who come from cultures that endorse high religiosity, even if the individuals don't subscribe to it themselves, have to contend with these religious shame-based cultural recipes, but that doesn't seem to be the case for people who identify as spiritual.

STRATEGIES FOR SACRED, SANCTIFIED SEX

Sex can be a deeply spiritual experience, and different religions offer perspectives on how to find that connection. Abrahamic religions, like Christianity, Islam, and Judaism, have texts that celebrate aspects of sexual pleasure and intimacy. The Song of Solomon in the Bible is a prime example. While some patriarchal views exist within these religions, there's also recognition of mutuality, like the Torah's acknowledgment of a woman's right to enjoyable sex. Additionally, progressive religious leaders are emerging, like Muslim sexologist Angelica Lindsey-Ali and Christian sexologist Brittany Broaddus-Smith. Following such voices can help you navigate your faith and have a fulfilling sex life. However, religious institutions may not always be the most forthcoming about sex. If that's the case, there are other paths to explore spiritual sex. Consider seeking guidance from spiritual teachers within your chosen tradition or finding books and online resources that explore the intersection of sexuality and spirituality. These resources can help you find a way to connect intimacy with your spiritual beliefs.

For people seeking spiritual sex outside of the more common religious traditions, there are many considerations and options. First, spiritual sex is not meant to create the feeling of shame. It is designed to remind you of connectedness with whatever you perceive as a higher power or omnipotence. Imagine engaging in sex with a sense of empowerment, rather than fear of upsetting a mean-ass god. Second, spiritual sex is also a reminder that you're connected to everything. It honors interdependence, such that everything from the natural environment is also meaningfully connected to you. The people Puritans once called witches—mostly women and gender expansive people; people who engage in marginalized spiritual practices like voodoo, Santeria, and other Indigenous spiritualities; and people of the global majority—were burned because they accessed these powers. You might imagine, as I do, that people already enacting social dominance and power—mostly land-owning white men—wouldn't just create a concerted effort to burn people who aren't harnessing something meaningful and empowering. There may be something to sex magic.

History tells us that sexually marginalized and gender expansive people had wisdom and a connection to the divine that most precolonial cultures respected. They established sexual rituals that honored bodies, nature, time, souls, and how they're all connected. Each culture had, and many still have, rituals unique to them.

One approach to spiritual sex is to research what your ancestors did. Start with more credible sources like Google Scholar to find historical books, but if you're following creators tapped into precolonial histories in your cultures, their guidance will be invaluable. There are many things that do not get into scholastic archives because, well, they're sacred. So the scholars you read should care about the cultural and spiritual histories you study, and that wasn't the case with many ethnographers, anthropologists, and historians of the past. Many were invested in misrepresenting cultures foreign to them, judging them through limited lenses to give themselves a sense of self-importance. They were also beholden to authorities that didn't want to reflect the nuance and attributes of people their governments and capitalists wanted to colonize. Basically, literate white men in Europe and early America had a vested interest in maligning spiritual sexual practices adopted by people who were different from them in any way. Being such a global minority, they were likely scared, so they were doing what scared men in power do: make up fantasies and myths to make themselves feel better, then coerce other people into believing them.

Shout out to the Haitian Vodou practitioners, New Orleans voo-doo queens, and other Afro-Indigenous people who were resilient enough to hold onto their spiritual traditions through the violence of the Transatlantic slave trade and colonialism. A lot of their practices were misrepresented in the movies and even more recently co-opted for capitalism, but they offer a template in how to harness and sustain the power of your spiritual heritage as resistance and as an avenue to good sex.

Once you find a book or old document from your cultural heritage that speaks to your spiritual beliefs, find out what spiritual sex means from that lens. Even if it is one that aligns with the historical and contemporary status quo, consider ways to make that practice more intentional. For example, if you align with Christianity, read Song of Solomon and establish a beautiful sexual experience that may include lilies, oils, and absolute reverence expressed through poetry for your lover. Or, if you want to learn more about Santeria, look to the queer practitioners who are often teachers of the practice for guidance. Engage in one spiritual practice from whatever tradition speaks to you for two months and journal about how your spiritual framework is impacting your sex life. Use the framework from earlier in this chapter to highlight the components of spirituality that mean the most to you, as your guide.

Sincere covered a lot of ground quickly because she had done a lot of historical work on the spiritual sexual practices of her tribe. In fact, her asexuality felt so at home to her because she had the critical consciousness to explain how it further grounded her in a decolonized version of her spiritual heritage. For her, good sex wasn't about engaging in sexual acts with others but becoming one of the elders who could share sexual wisdom with people going through various age-based rites of passage. She hosted sessions for the preteens who were to begin menstruating or experiencing nocturnal emission, which were basically culturally relevant, comprehensive, sex-positive, sex education courses. They could ask her the things they were embarrassed or scared to ask their parents, and the parents relied on her expertise and comfort discussing sexual subjects. Many of the parents acknowledged how they still felt awkward talking about sex, and they were more comfortable letting her talk about it because of, not despite, her asexuality.

Sincere also provided teaching for the people who felt ready to make their sexual debuts, people experiencing hormone imbalances that led to sexual dysfunction, and people dealing with infertility. She taught other ace community members about the vastness and divinity of asexuality as an identity and as a valuable community role. She wondered with the Christians, "What if Jesus was ace, rather than abstinent?" Many of them became her protégés so that the wisdom of spiritual sex could live on once she transitioned to the ancestors.

Her teachings, while initially unsettling to some traditionalists, eventually found fertile ground. Even conservative members softened as they faced life's realities—changing bodies, fading intimacy, and the loss of connection with loved ones due to rigid societal norms. Through her work as a spiritual sex mentor, she fostered a profound sense of community care and repair. Sincere even established a dedicated lodge, a sacred space where people could reconnect with the divine through sexual exploration. In her own words, she saw herself as a conduit, allowing the Spirit to flow through her and become a source of sexual well-being for her community. This act of selfless service cemented her legacy as a revolutionary figure among her tribe, one who dared to bridge the gap between sexuality and spirituality.

13

Good Sex
is Sensual

At a basic, biochemical level, sensuality is like electricity, and I've lost some of mine. Something in my body's circuit system doesn't seem to allow me to conduct energy like I once did. It was a gradual loss, easy to overlook in the demands of being a tenure track professor, then a wife, then a mom, all within the context of reproductive health challenges, grief, and the pandemic. It's something writing this book is helping me recover, but it is important to highlight that even as a sex researcher and therapist, even as someone who believes in her own pleasure-worthiness, I am not exempt from the human experience. I'm not the final boss of good sex. I'm practicing it with you. Sensuality is a core part of the practice.

When my now husband and I met, I was exploring spiritual traditions like Buddhism and A Course in Miracles. I'd even explored Quakerism after taking a spirituality quiz to see what might best align with my intuitive spiritual leanings. I was spiritually questioning and quite open to possibilities that helped me feel peace, joy, and love. He was trying to deepen his spiritual walk through Christianity, and he was hoping for a partner—a wife—that wanted to walk that path with him. I wanted to be a wife so badly, assuming it would give me the peace, joy, and love (value and purpose) I was looking for, that I chose Christianity again. As a sign of my commitment, I suggested we abstain from any more sex until we were married. We got married eleven months later. While those eleven months strengthened our friendship (something I value), the abstinence, coupled with certain interpretations of Christian ideals we adopted, ultimately hindered our sexual intimacy.

There were also the reproductive health challenges, which began in my midtwenties, during the first years of my doctoral training. I had symptomatic uterine fibroids. Their growth led to excessive menstrual bleeding, resulting in anemia and fatigue, as well as several embarrassing accidents and an obsession with naturally resolving the symptoms that never worked. I didn't experience relief until I was in my midthirties following multiple surgeries. Until then, I felt my body was attacking itself. I was in a womb war, and my sensual self was unknowingly wounded as well.

During that time, I lost my aunt Tonja, a key maternal figure who gave me permission to be a fast Black girl and a sensual Black woman, to a vegetative state following a fatal asthma attack. This occurred in the same year I had begun my dream job as a professor. I got seduced by the overwork that was such a welcome reprieve from my grief. And I started drinking wine more regularly, even though I hadn't really been a drinker up until then.

We welcomed our first child in 2019, which again reoriented my relationship to my body, sensuality, and my sexual self. Then, COVID-19 hit alongside the 2020 racial reckoning. With some of my work being in healing racial trauma, I again opted into overwork to meet the demands of what I felt at the time was my contribution to the resistance. By 2021, conservative groups and media had maligned my work, intentionally misrepresenting me as a person who believed white people were inferior to other people, when in fact I taught the crux of oppressive behavior is the oppressor's failure to recognize their shared and equal humanity with all humans. Exacerbating the stress and trauma of an already trying year, that summer I experienced an ectopic pregnancy where my fallopian tube burst and nearly killed me. I didn't trust my body to enjoy good sex, or even sensual pleasure, for the rest of that summer. It was easier to simply be numb, to unconsciously hit the off switch on the remaining electricity I used to enjoy.

I share these key moments because most of us have these hallmark times when things obviously shifted in our sensuality. And it isn't just the moments of distress and trauma that divorce us from our sensuality. It's also the way we understand those moments through the most pervasive sexual cultural recipes that limit our ability to use the good sex ingredients. What I had unknowingly internalized was an idea that being numb, not feeling anything at all, could protect me from physical and emotional pain. It's a common belief because it is partially true. If you're having a tooth extracted, you want to be temporarily numb. Novocain protects you from pain, but you also can't feel your mouth or taste anything while it is active. This is fine for the immediacy of the extraction and the first few days of recovery, but numbing through overwork, substance use, binge eating (binge anything, really), suppresses your sensuality.

Health issues and medical trauma, purity culture, patriarchy, capitalism, elitism, gendered racism, global syndemic, and grief all too effectively snuffed out my sensuality.

VOLUPTUOUS PLEASURES: SENSIBLE V. SENSUAL

There was a divide in the cultural recipes that uplifted being sensible and denigrated being sensual around the fifteenth century. Though the words come from the same word root, European moralists asserted that there was something superior about being logical, practical, and mentally astute, and something base and vulgar about enjoying the senses of sight, sound, touch, taste, and smell. *Sensual*'s early definitions of "endowed with feeling" and "carnal, of the body" present embodiment as lewd, unchaste, devoted to voluptuous pleasures. I, for one, think voluptuous pleasures sound amazing; however, the Europeans, partaking in them nonetheless, at least wanted to put on the record that they were above having a good time.

As discussed in the fun chapter, creating a human hierarchy with whoever likes to enjoy themselves at the bottom persists today, even in a world where Adrienne Maree Brown's *Pleasure Activism* exists. Brown calls readers in to get sensual and explore some of the options to feel and experience pleasure again. But the constant demands of daily life can leave us feeling disconnected from our bodies, or we feel so deeply that we opt out through numbing, which benefits oppression rather than humans. Ivan Brady says, "Human beings are sensual and intellectual creatures," not one or the other. The lack of somatic awareness, or body awareness, makes it difficult to connect with our sensuality and enjoy good sex.

By now, it's clear that sex is more than simply a physical touch experience. The way we feel, think, and contextualize sex are important, but the way we sense sex goes beyond touch. Unfortunately, the same intersectional oppression that blocks us from other good sex ingredients is at work in our sensual selves. This is largely because the sensual has been in located in people of the global majority's bodies, especially women. And since women of the global majority's bodies occupy a marginalized place in society, sensuality itself becomes marginalized too.

THE SCIENCE OF SENSES

Remember the five senses we learned about in grade school—sight, sound, smell, taste, and touch? Science tells us these senses work through electrical signals. Take hearing, for example. Sound waves vibrate the eardrum, triggering tiny hair cells in the cochlea. These hair cells convert the vibrations into electrical signals that travel to the brain, where they're interpreted as sound.

This electrical dance within us is key to understanding sensuality. Hearing a favorite sex song creates a positive emotional connection—the electrical impulses from hearing the music become associated with the pleasant mood you feel. These positive associations, along with those from other senses, can be amplified or dampened, influencing how we experience sensuality. That's why my research team started our meetings with a different team member's favorite sex song each week, and why we opted to ask our research participants what their favorite sex songs were too. We created the Big Sex Study playlist as a sensual intervention. Songs can even hint toward what someone may desire sexually. Destin Mizelle led our study on Black men's favorite sex songs and found that R&B was their favorite genre, they almost equally enjoyed songs that focused on mutual, partner, and self-pleasure, and the song topics focused on "attentiveness and admiration of partner, fulfilling fantasy, lust and yearning, vocal affirmation and reassurance, casual and concurrent sex partners, and desire for intimacy." So, in addition to the sensual nature of the type of melodies from the R&B genre, the words also spoke to auditory pleasure as sensual.

As another example, smell was the most definitive determinant above the other senses for cis women choosing a sexual partner. For cis men, visual and smell were equal. Rachel Herz and Elizabeth Cahill compared sight, hearing, touch, and smell for sexual arousal too.

During sex, men ranked sight and touch—how their partner looks and feels to them—as most likely to arouse them than the other senses. Notably, music was their lowest ranked source of arousal. Women also ranked touch highest, sight was second (not as high as it was for men), and body smells lowest. In a nonsexual context, how their partner looks was the most likely to arouse men and women. So different senses have appeal given the context. Mindfulness can help you attune to whichever senses appeal most to you.

STRATEGIES FOR SENSUAL SEX: SLOW THE F*CK DOWN

Sensual sex requires most people to move a little slower or spend a bit of extra time to be sure the senses are engaged. Because most of us are numb or otherwise distracted, we're still taking in sensory information, but we're less able to appreciate it. Mindful attention is not rushed, so you'll likely need to slow the fuck down, in every way I can mean that, to enjoy sensual sex.

Because sight is a sense that increases the chances that sex will be good, second highest to touch, being mindful about how you and your partner look is one way to enhance sensual sex. If you want to focus on partnered sensual sex, ask each other what look is most appealing. Wearing a certain outfit, shaving your beard a certain way, being oiled up, putting on certain lip colors may all be visual sensual arousal cues. Even the act of intentionally grooming can be sensual. So the next three times you have sex, each of you can go for the look your partner desires and gauge how much you enjoy the sexual experience. For some people, a T-shirt and panties may be a visually appealing look (shout out to Adina Howard). For others, gray sweatpants may do it. It's me. I'm others. Some partners may want more intentionally sexy clothes like lingerie. If you're having solo sex, groom and dress yourself in a way that appeals to you.

For both men and women, being able to focus on touch/feeling is primary when it comes to sex. My favorite sensual sex practice for enhancing touch is sensate focus. For those of you who have a wandering mind, are easily prone to boredom, or are hyperkinetic—have a difficult time being still—this can be especially helpful. As a derivative of sensate focus, which is a sex therapy technique to help couples who are experiencing sexual dysfunction, you can use the touch options with partners or alone. You can spend ten to thirty minutes touching your partner in nongenital areas intentionally with different forms of pressure, friction, vibration, and temperature. The point isn't to initiate sexual arousal, although if that happens, it's no problem at all. The point is to engage your sense of touch and theirs. Doing the touching and being touched are both useful. Being nude together while you enjoy this activity can make it more intimate. For a clinical version of sensate focus, work with a licensed professional, but simply taking fifteen minutes to intentionally, mindfully touch each other twice a week can be a good start for simply enhancing sensual sex.

Haptic communication is how we speak nonverbally through touch. Consider what messages you send your partner and yourself, based on how you touch your body. What messages do you want to send? Now, other senses can be brought in to enhance the sensuality of the experience. For example, light a candle that smells enticing, play a song that sounds soothing or write your lover a poem that you read them, make sure the space you're in looks visually appealing, and even think about whether you see yourself as visually appealing. Also, the introduction of a simple food—honey, chocolate, berries—may further engage the senses.

Finally, reduce your use of things that numb you out. If you typically drink three glasses of wine at the end of a day, drink one instead. If you typically use work to tune out of life, allow yourself to take fifteen-minute breaks after seventy-five minutes of work time, even if it means dealing with the normal, human pain that comes alongside the joy of living. If you typically spend more minutes or hours than you would like scrolling social media or binge watching TV, choose to do a set amount of time. This is a harm reduction approach, rather than an abstinence approach. Abstinence would require you to forgo the things that may become or already have become numbing agents for you.

Learning mindful moderation, rather than abstinence, is a more accessible approach to mindfully reengaging your sensuality. In fact, I suspect some people use abstinence as another form of numbing, through self-deprivation. For example, if I had to do it again, I may have learned some valuable lessons about sex, my religious journey, and my romantic relationship had my husband and I not opted to abstain for nearly a year. Practices like yoga, including the stretches and meditation, can also help you return to your senses.

During that period of nearly a decade where I struggled most with my sensuality, I started a program called Sensations. I started it for myself, but I also wanted other women in my community to participate. The program had a series of yoga-based stretches that we held while listening to sensual music, then we did erotic choreography for the remainder of the class. It lasted about one semester, but I did notice the benefits for myself. Frankly, I'm terrible at marketing, so I didn't always have people show up for the class, but I committed to doing it whether someone came or not. My body felt more responsive to touch, the essential oil diffuser had the studio smelling amazing, and I was listening to music I enjoyed regularly. Just addressing those three of five senses was a great start. I stopped due to surgery, but it's something I want to restart.

Now, I'm in the daily practice of reclaiming sensual life moments so they can translate to my sexual experiences. When I notice I'm eating fast, I slow down and seek to savor the taste. I make sure my home, office, and car smell incredibly good. I have sensual playlists and erotic audiostories that I listen to with music that moves me. These practices are helping me return home to my sensual self, reacquaint with my body and how it perceives the world around it, and open myself up to good sex. As a mom (writing this exact sentence with a newborn on my lap), I'm admittedly not taking the time to look sensually appealing. I have self-compassion and am okay with that at this stage of breastfeeding, C-section recovery, and interrupted sleep, but I look forward to getting back to it. I enjoy writing this chapter while I'm still toying with aspects of my practice, because as I'm synthesizing the research to develop strategies for others, I'm doing the same for me.

14

Good Sex
is Communicative

Date one was an ice cream date, chocolate with sprinkles for Will, butter pecan for Malcolm. Malcolm shared, "My grandma, who basically raised me, always had some butter pecan in the freezer. It was her favorite, so eating it is how I stay close to her now that she's gone. This is the only ice cream shop I know of that still sells it." Will touched Malcolm's cheekbone, as a tear rolled down it. They hadn't even kissed, but he was falling in love.

Date two was dinner. Will shared, "My family runs a Korean barbeque restaurant back home in Cali. Since we lived in a college town, we had so many kinds of people coming in and trying our culture. I like sharing it with you." While they flirted over their dinner, Will carefully pulled a piece of beef off the grill, blew on it, then fed it to Malcolm. Malcolm said, "See, I can get with Korean food, because y'all know how to season your meat." They laughed, and he fell in love.

By date three, both Will and Malcolm had gotten used to talking on the phone every night and sending cute wake up texts each morning. They were holding hands on the way back to the car from the movie theater when Will said, "I've got to tell you something, especially since I'm really feeling you."

Malcolm opened his car door, let Will get in, then walked as slowly as possible to the driver's side to catch his breath. No good conversation ever started with "I've got to tell you something."

Inside the car, Will's heartbeat had doubled. He was holding his breath, noticing how slowly Malcolm was walking. He exhaled a little when Malcolm finally opened the door and got in. Malcolm had decided in his slow walk that if Will said anything out of pocket, he was going to take him straight home and never call him again.

"So, what is it you have to tell me?"

"I feel some fear letting you know, but I would rather be transparent. I'm really feeling you, and I want to take it to the next level, so honest communication is important to me." He paused. "I have HSV."

Malcolm busted out laughing. "Boy, I thought you was finna tell me something terrible. Shit, who don't have herpes these days? But thank you for telling me before we had sex." He laughed some more.

Will felt the humor rise along with the relief. "So, you're just gonna laugh at me in my face," he said, trying to hold back his own laughter.

"I like you too. I want to, how did you say it, take it to the next level too. Sounding like an episode of Saved by the Bell. Of course, I'm laughing."

They laughed together, solidifying the start of their open communication. On the way home, they talked about what they liked sexually, how they could get their sexual needs met if the other wasn't interested, and different kinks they wanted to try, and ending in one of the best nights of sex either had ever had.

EXPRESSIVE AND RECEPTIVE COMMUNICATION

Early definitions of *communicate* from the 1500s related to sharing information or a feeling. Beyond facts being transmitted, what we say and how we say it can invoke emotional and somatic experiences. Sexual communication is important before, during, and after sex, but the types of communication may differ at the various time points. Verbal, assertive, and direct communication are typically privileged above other forms because they offer the clearest indication of what the communicator is hoping to convey. Now, the saying that nonverbal accounts for 93 percent of how we communicate has been proven to be a myth, but it is worth noting that actions, gestures, and tone are valid sources of communication too. If I shake my head side to side when someone asks if I like something, they can typically assume I mean no. That's also why conversations related to consent are important and need to happen more often and in more nuanced ways. The "no means no" era ignored the many other ways one can say no without those words.

Sexual communication is a way of letting your partner know what makes sex good for you, in whatever way you define that. When the communication is open and flowing back and forth, the reward is a sexual partner who doesn't have to guess. And there's a difference between guessing someone's wants/needs and being curious about them. Curious people ask questions. Guessers usually assume without asking. Sexual communication leads to increased sexual satisfaction and pleasure, less sexual harm and pain, and improved chances of cultivating intimacy. But if we know these are the benefits of sexual communication, why is it so hard?

We live in a world where only some people are expected to be the expressive communicators—the ones who talk or send the message. Those of us who are multiply marginalized are often required to be the receptive communicators—the listeners. So, because we live in a patriarchal, racist, classist, sexist, heterosexist—I could go on—society, people with multiple marginalized identities are expected to listen carefully. For example, most heterosexual relationship cultural recipes expect the woman to be the better listener. There are many stereotypes about men being poor communicators, when all genders are equally as capable of developing these skills. If you're a man with good communication skills, many people respond to you as if you're an anomaly, and in some circles, there is a hidden script that it's unmanly to be a good listener.

This perceived gap in listening may be relevant to the pleasure and orgasm gap in sex. That is, if you're unable or unwilling to listen to what your partner desires, it is less likely you'll be able to help them experience good sex. Most studies show that everything from orgasm and arousal to overall sexual functioning are improved by good quality sexual communication, so how well you communicate does matter. Communication is also about being able to tell your person what you want, and some studies suggest cis women find that more difficult than men. Women don't want to be perceived as bossy, ungrateful, too eager, or hypersexual, so they may avoid essential conversations early on. It then becomes harder to initiate the conversations the longer they wait. However, there isn't clear evidence on how balanced sexual communication is among trans or non-binary people.

Sexual communication is key to not only enhancing pleasure (chapter 3) but also practicing safer sex. However, discussing condoms, birth control, sexually transmitted infections (STIs), desires for children or not, and consent can be difficult for many people. Power dynamics can make these conversations even trickier. That is what made Will so afraid to tell Malcolm about his HSV. In the past, partners had tried to shame him about it. Sure, communication skills are important, but skill alone can't overcome fear, social pressures, or the potential for negative consequences. The receptive listener has to also have the capacity to listen with care. Sex education programs often miss the mark by focusing solely on communication skills without acknowledging the context. Communication needs to be honest, welcomed, and a two-way street, because a study by Uzma Rehman and colleagues reports that three main types of barriers to communication are:

- **Threats to Self:** fear that communication can evoke shame, guilt, embarrassment, or other uncomfortable feelings; fear of looking sexually inadequate by revealing a lack of sexual skill or experience; fear of limited communication skills.

- **Threats to Partner:** fear of hurting or making the partner uncomfortable; fear of evoking distrust or low self-esteem in the partner.

- **Threats to Relationship:** fear that the romantic relationship will be less stable following communication due to revealed incompatibility, beliefs that talking about certain topics should not be necessary, or beliefs that talking about issues makes them worse.

They found that people are more likely to experience threats to self during conflicts about sex versus other topics. So simply teaching communication skills is only one step. It is necessary to address the perceived threats felt when broaching sexual communication and fight against relationship recipes that punish open communication unfairly. Finally, we should create or improve systems that encourage open, honest, caring, and courageous conversations about sex. Valerie Rubinsky and Angela M. Hosek suggest LGBTQ people are likely better prepared for sexual communication because they have had to be more forthcoming in sexual self-disclosure earlier and more often. This is perhaps why Will, despite fearing potential threats to his budding relationship with Malcolm and threats to self, still courageously disclosed his STI status early on in their dating.

STRATEGIES FOR SEXUAL COMMUNICATION: COMMUNICATING THE GOOD AND BAD

Most people assume that sexual communication is only relevant when there is an issue, but the biggest way to reduce the three threats and increase the quality of sexual communication is to communicate about the good and the bad. When you and your partner(s) make it a point to talk about sex positively, your communication comfort increases. So the Yes, No, Maybe So activity shared in chapter 3 provides an opportunity to talk about what you like in a low stakes manner. Additionally, letting your partner know when something they did feels good during or after sexual experiences is another way to make sexual communication a normal, balanced element of your relationship.

That said, broaching more taboo, stigmatized, or conflict-laden sexual topics is still necessary. Returning to the Yes, No, Maybe So activity, communication skills and contexts are important. Consider if you shared your list with a new partner, and they "yucked your yum," a term sex educators use to discourage shaming other people's sexual preferences and desires just because they don't align with yours. Their shaming communication, whether a facial expression or a disgusted utterance, can make you feel less incentivized to share more. If this is someone you really like, even more so. But your communication skill can be a corrective. Namely, if you have the skill to let them know that you felt shamed when they responded that way, and you're looking for the type of sexual experience where shaming isn't a part of it, they can now become more aware of their behavior (intended or not) and opt to change or learn something new with you. But if you shut down, it's more likely they'll never know how you felt hurt and miss out on some potentially good sexual experiences you could share. Honestly, most people get somewhat stuck in this.

Another communication barrier is hoping people just guess your sexual preferences and desires, to avoid the vulnerability of having to communicate them. It takes courage to ask for what you want, and sometimes we impose the "mindreading" script on our partners because we think they're just supposed to know. There are some partners who are more intuitive or observant than others, but even that is a skill learned over time. If you're already aware your sexual partner doesn't have that strength, then communicating with them what you want, almost as many times as you want it, will be the best option. For some people, having to communicate makes it less valuable (relationship threat); they think it means more when the offering is organic. Remember, changing a behavior takes time and effort. It won't happen as quickly as you might wish.

MEANINGFUL METACOMMUNICATION

Metacommunication is another strategy that may be helpful. It's what happens when you talk about how you're communicating. Use the three sexual communication threats as your framework. First, assess which threats are most salient for you and why. It could be one or all of them. This may be something you journal about or discuss together. Do this before you're in a conflict or have a need to discuss a sexual subject. Next, when you do want to have a sexual conversation, you can let your partner(s) know which threats may be activated. For example, you could say, "I'm afraid our relationship might be shakier after I say this, and I don't want that, but I want honesty more than I want to avoid talking." You can also let your sexual partner know that "When

I feel sad, it's harder for me to talk things through, but my face may look like this. It would help me if you initiate a conversation if you see me looking sad." In this way, you offer them a way to pick up on your nonverbal communication cues well before they need to. Similarly, you can say, "Sometimes I get aroused, get hard, even when I'm not in the mood. It's important to me that you know I'll tell you explicitly if I want to be sexual. Don't use my body as your guide, because it seems to have a mind of its own."

It's important to remember that metacommunication is an ongoing process, not a one-time fix. As you and your partner continue to grow and change, your needs and preferences will likely evolve as well. So be prepared to have regular conversations about how you're communicating and what you're each feeling. This will help you stay on the same page and ensure that your sexual relationship remains satisfying for both of you.

On the flip side, if you're more attuned to picking up on cues, you can voice your observations and ask if they align with your partner's true feelings. This nips assumptions in the bud, which can often snowball into stories your mind conjures up based on your deepest anxieties. For instance, if your partner seems animated and chatty, you could say, "You seem energized by our playful interaction. Is that how you're feeling?" This opens the door for them to either confirm your intuition or offer a different perspective. It also helps them become more aware of what they might be projecting and what you're perceiving. Remember, clear communication is a two-way street, and both partners need to be willing to express themselves honestly and listen attentively to build a truly fulfilling sexual connection.

Just like any other language, metacommunication takes practice. It's not always about grand pronouncements or emotional outpourings. Sometimes, the most important metacommunication happens in the quiet moments in between. A knowing glance, a gentle touch, or a playful nudge can all be ways of communicating your desires and needs to your partner without saying a word. The key is to be attuned to your partner's nonverbal cues and to use your own body language to send clear and positive messages.

Because many people are shamed for talking about sex, or experience negative consequences in their relationships for giving sexual feedback, we also need to address how the ego can become involved in communicative sex. When you have not been taught how to talk about sex most of your life AND many people—especially men and masculine-of-center people—derive part of their sense of value from their sexual prowess, telling someone the sex is not yet good can be difficult. Many women and feminine-of-center people have accepted scripts that they are out of order for communicating with men and masculine-of-center people about their sexual needs, especially in the moment. That being good at sex is tied to ego is the problem, not the communication of sexual desires. People think you're calling them, rather than their sexual skill set, inadequate. No one likes to feel that way, even if that wasn't the intent of the communication.

I appreciate this generation of women in hip-hop who use their songs to highlight how to communicate about sex with a partner, but even they miss the mark when they shift the communication from information to degradation. Can you tell someone that a position is painful, that you don't want your pussy beat up, and still feel secure? Can you do it in a way that honors they may have been doing what they know best, rather than assuming the worst? Can they receive feedback without feeling humiliated and withdrawing or lashing out? Healthier sexual partners can broach sexual communication with care and receive sexual communication without defensiveness. Depending on what your reasons for having sex were, it may be better to end things with a partner who can't accept your carefully provided sexual feedback or provide it in a caring way than to stop communicating all together.

WRITING AND ROLE-PLAY

It can be easier for some people to write their communication down than speak it. Some people can speak it better than they can show it. Some people can show you better than they can tell you. Each of these ways of sexually communicating are valid, but you want to know which one you and your sexual partner(s) tend to use most, so you can be aware of where to focus your attention. What way is it easier for you to communicate? Which one comes most naturally to you, and which communication styles do you need to work on a bit more? Ask your sexual partner to answer these questions too. Provide examples from your own relationship dynamic if you can, so they can know what it looked like when communication was easy or hard.

Role-plays can contribute to good sex in many ways, but I don't mean the Little Red Riding Hood/Big Bad Wolf variety in this case. In this instance, I mean role-playing the type of sexual communication that works for you before you need to do the communicating. First, do an animated role-play of yourself and how you communicate with your partner. Articulate the metacommunication, what your ego is saying, and how you would communicate in a specific scenario of their choosing. Then, have your partner do the same. Get as over the top as possible and be willing to laugh at yourselves. This will bring levity to the topic of sexual communication, which we sometimes take too seriously.

Then, both of you write out a script for how you want to communicate the same things. The script writing process, with edits and all, can help you overcome the difficulty of having to think extemporaneously. You get edits in your script that you aren't always afforded in life. Looking at how you wrote it the first time, you may notice that you hedged on your actual sexual needs in a way that didn't really convey your desires. You can revise it. Then, practice those edited scripts with each other more than once. The first time is to learn how to say it and get the jitters out. The second and third time are to own it and let it really land with your partner. Even though you are both simply acting out the scenarios, there are things you want each other to know that still ring true as you each listen to each other.

Then, solicit feedback on the delivery. Did you experience your partner's role-play as assertive, kind, loving, or whatever way you prefer to be communicated with? How did they experience your tone, nonverbals, and verbals? Were there things missing that your partner wants more clarity on? These questions can help both of you refine your communication styles and content. Ultimately, the goal is to practice saying what you mean, without being mean with what you say.

I don't say everything I'm thinking to avoid saying things I don't mean. Just because something pops into my head doesn't mean it's ready to share with the world. Thoughts are like rough drafts—they need time and refinement before they become something others need to hear. What I speak or write down is a better reflection of the message I want to deliver than the thought I had. And some thoughts, I recognize, aren't healthy for me or my partner. As a person in the practice of healing, thoughts may occasionally reflect some of the wounded parts that are seeking to wound others. Process that in therapy or in a journal.

Malcolm and Will had solid communication going for them most of the time. The fact that they could be honest, vulnerable, and light with each other helped set the stage for the times when the attachment differences felt a bit overwhelming and got in the way. They had a history of good communication that they returned to in therapy, and we were able to use that to repair many sexual disagreements.

"Remember, y'all, you're the couple who laughed while you were sharing a positive STI status. You're made of the stuff that can stand the test of time," I offered.

"You're right. Because I will never forget him laughing in my face when I told him. It let me know I could laugh and be a little lighter too," Will said.

So, using a little psychodrama, we spent the rest of that session doing sexual communication role-play, ego style. By the end of it, Malcolm was standing up clapping hands, rolling his neck, fully expressing the major fear he felt before Will disclosed his STI. Will was laughing so hard his stomach hurt. Then he also got into character and communicated what he was feeling too, giving the performance of a lifetime. We used a communication scene they already went through positively to help them learn role-play skills, so they could apply them to other conflicts as they arose.

15

Good Sex
is Wet

I didn't like Cardi B and Megan Thee Stallion's "WAP" . . . at first. The "There's some hoes in this house" sample immediately took me back to the Armory in Franklin, Virginia, around 1997, where on any given party night I could be found in the middle of the dance floor encircled by encouraging peers while a friend and I pussy popped in a split. Shout out to Frank Ski and Al "T" McLaran for that early '90s hit that made my youth vibrant. But by August 2020, amid the pandemic and the 2020 racial reckoning, I was thirty-seven years old and shut in with my husband and a one-year-old son, tired of everyone and everything, and having a hard time finding my joy. The last thing I was thinking of, even as a sex researcher, was how to make my pussy wetter. At that time, it seemed like maybe my natural lubrication, which had been a beautiful, abundant feature of my twenties and early thirties, may never return. Resigned, I was focused on healing racial trauma and cultivating anti-racism. I had forgotten that without a more comprehensive definition of liberation, one that included joy and pleasure for me too, the ability to enjoy wetness and other good sex ingredients might remain compromised.

WET, WETTER, WETTEST

Natural lubrication—the viscous fluid that moisturizes the vaginal walls and opening—is only one of many indicators of sexual arousal for people with vaginas. As you may recall from earlier chapters, arousal is different from desire. It's your body's way of indicating preparedness to make a sexual experience easier and potentially more pleasurable. But the cultural recipes on being wet, wetter, wettest that I navigate as a Black woman have an interesting history. Qualifying the amount of natural lubrication someone creates is just another way we reinforce a human hierarchy based on perceived desirability, ableism, and the patriarchal centering of penetrative sex over all forms of sex.

Tee Noir from the same-named YouTube channel does one of the best analyses of this topic in her video essay "Hypersexuality and the Perfect Pussy Complex," so I want to bring a few of her points home here. Sexual lubrication is a sign of vaginal and sexual health, but using natural sexual lubrication as a barometer of your worthiness as a sexual partner is not conducive to good sex. Wetness gets wrapped up in standards of womanliness, sexiness, genital grooming, to be of service to one's partner, rather than a signal to yourself that maybe your sexual capacity is shifting or hindered due to aging, lack of interest, dehydration, sexual dysfunction, or not enough foreplay.

Hip-hop plays a major role in promoting the idea that a woman's sexual value is based on how wet she gets. This focus on lubrication as a measure of arousal is a recent addition to the bravado found in hip-hop lyrics. Traditionally, rappers have competed by boasting about material possessions (money, cars, clothes) and even sexual conquests. Now, being the wettest woman has become another way to claim superiority. In many ways it can feel like a corrective to the constant dehumanization many Black people face. However, it can also be argued that it reinforces negative stereotypes about Black sexuality, rather than freeing Black women from those expectations. The allure of dominance is undeniable. It's exciting to see Black women asserting themselves in hip-hop, and I admire artists like Cardi B, Glorilla, and Megan Thee Stallion for their brand of hip hop feminism. However, it's important to acknowledge that even positive expressions can have unintended consequences.

WAP can be a good thing, but it won't always come naturally to everyone with a vagina, and that doesn't make them less valuable or desirable. We know for sure that bussies—or anuses—another area where people may be penetrated, require adequate, externally applied lubrication. Why would we hold people with vaginas to a higher standard of ability to get wet on demand, effortlessly, when many options of purchasable lubrication exist? Patriarchy.

Culturally, not everyone is into WAP. I was surprised and thoroughly interested in learning that there are some African sexual traditions that prioritize dry sex, and women in those cultures use astringent agents vaginally to create the dry experience. Notably, this can increase vaginal tearing and irritation, as well as the potential for contracting STIs. This norm promotes another unrealistic and harmful belief that women with "tighter" vaginas are more desirable or moral, which is simply not true. However, in the typical USA context, the combination of both tight and wet are commonly lauded.

LUBE LITERACY

A 2010 paper entitled "The Ins and Outs of Vaginal Lubrication," interestingly written by a male sexual functioning scholar Roy J. Levin, describes the process of lubrication. When something turns you on—whether it's a thought, a touch, a picture, or a sound—your brain gets a message that something exciting is about to happen, kind of like a preview for a fun movie. Because your body wants a 4D movie experience, blood flows to the vaginal canal and surrounding membranes through the blood vessels. The arousal function temporarily traps the blood there by making the blood vessels smaller. This constriction presses upon the various glands in the vagina, causing secretions that are beyond the normal "just moist enough to not have the vagina tissue atrophy and stick together" condition inside the vagina. This fluid feels less watery or tacky, and more slippery. That means it is better able to facilitate friction in a pleasurable or less painful way when something penetrates the vagina. But it isn't enough to get the vaginal walls wet in this way. Since the interior labia (labia minora) often cover the vaginal opening, producing or using enough lubrication to wet them is essential too. The labia, as it turns out, also produce lubrication when one is aroused.

As a reminder here, arousal does not indicate consent or sexual desire. It's simply the body's attempt to make sex more pleasurable and less painful should the person becoming aroused want to engage in sex.

Levin's description was as sound as he could make it based on the science at that time. He admits that most research has not been able to objectively measure vaginal lubrication well, because the main method to do so was sticking a dry tampon in the vagina, initiating arousal, and then taking the moistened tampon out to weigh it. You cannot do that multiple times in a row to measure different stages of arousal, because tampons wick away at the vaginal lining and cause irritation if used too frequently. To all my tampon users, recall that final day of your period when you realize the period is over because pulling out the dry tampon tells you so.

Newer research by Ariel Handy and Cindy Meston offers up additional ways to measure vaginal lubrication, as one of two aspects of arousal described above: blood flow and lubrication. They note that how wet you think you are may differ dramatically from how wet you are. For example, you may have really wanted to have sex and felt aroused and ready, only to have a tough time with penetration because there wasn't enough natural lubrication to ease the passage. Other examples from research include having women watch something erotic and using litmus strips—a newer way scientists measure lubrication—only to find the self-reported wetness was less than what the test found. In their study, the women who had sexual dysfunction self-reported lower lubrication, even though it was the same amount as women who didn't have sexual dysfunction. Bodies provide us information, but sometimes they lie.

One thing that gets in the way is the idea that we're supposed to be more lubricated than we are, even if the amount is enough. That's the wetness imperative I described earlier. Another is that stigma related to using sexual health resources, from toys to lubricants, is pervasive. Most research suggests adding lube to the sexual experience increases sexual health by lowering discomfort and pain and increasing pleasure . . . that's for everyone involved. It's the way we've been taught to think about it that makes some of us feel shameful.

Natural lubrication and capacity to lubricate does change during different times of the menstrual cycle, at different stages in life (pre- and post-menopause), and for a host of other reasons related to sexual interest, changes in ability status, and variations in stress. Using two types of treatment, based on the intended impact, can help with the physical part, while some rescripting can help with the way we perceive it.

STRATEGIES FOR WET SEX: LUBE IS FOR EVERYONE

Lubricants are different from vaginal moisturizers. The former is typically for a specific sexual or penetrative experience, used immediately before and during by anyone regardless of gender. The latter is for daily use to restore the vaginal pH balance and prevent irritation due to daily, non-sex-related dryness. Two considerations for choosing the best lubricants and moisturizers for you are pH and osmolality—or how the chemicals in the lubes get into your body. Researchers recommend finding a body identical replacement for your lube.

If you're already using lubricants for sex, consider how they were introduced. Was it reluctantly or fearfully? Or were they introduced with excitement and curiosity? If you're not currently using lubes, is it because you don't feel you need them, or because you fear using them will mean something is wrong with you? Same questions for vaginal moisturizers. And I also want to acknowledge that in a thorough article related to both lubricants and moisturizers, they used the term "colonization of the vagina," which I can't unsee and which can have so many meanings based on this topic.

Next, consider that different lubricants serve unique purposes. There are three bases for most lubricants: water, oil, silicone.

- Water-based lubricants work well with sex and sex toys, absorb into the skin with less irritation, and clean up well.

- Oil-based lubricants last the longest due to their thickness, but they are harder to clean up and erode latex. They're most likely to cause irritation, but doctors occasionally still recommend oils like coconut oil.

- Silicone-based lubricants are the happy medium between water and oil in how long they last and their compatibility with condoms and clean up. They don't work with silicone toys, but glass toys work just fine.

The type of lubricant you need is based on the sexual situation, so feel free to buy a few options to try them out. If you're already someone who uses lubricants, trying new ones can help you expand your repertoire. If you're new to lube, this will help you secure your staple. There are so many ways to make good sex wet, and research suggests that water-based lubes are a good starting place. Try three brands for penetrative sex, giving each a three-peat before you move on to the next one. Journal about how the sex feels and whether the lubricant agrees with your genitalia. If none of them work well, try a few more.

Additionally, even though store bought lube is good for every sexual encounter, there still may be concern about your natural lubrication. As research indicates, some women and other people with vulvas may think they're less wet than they are; ask yourself what standard you may be comparing yourself to. Is it your previous lubrication capacity or a made-up idea? Then, consider the length of time you're engaging in foreplay, the stress level in your life, the time of the month, hormonal contraceptive use, medications, and where you're at within your reproductive life (pre-, peri-, or post-menopause). Additionally, consider your relationship quality. All of these can affect your ability to experience sexual arousal in general. As a starter experiment, try to increase the time you spend in the beginning of a sexual encounter by five to ten extra minutes. Try that for the next three sex sessions and see if your body responds to the extra attention.

I was introduced to lubricants by my college boyfriend in the early 2000s, as they were a typical part of his solo and partnered sexual routine. At that point, self-lubricating wasn't an issue, but I didn't mind trying something new. It was lovely to be introduced to them in a no-shame context, because as I began to need them after my midthirties, they were already in regular use. I realized that I needed them when the lube, on rare occasions, ran out, and I felt more discomfort and even some pain. My husband's size feels wonderful with, and not so wonderful without, added lube to me. But I began to feel some guilt and upset that my body just wasn't working the way it used to work, especially as someone who studies sex for a living.

The more I learned as a sex scientist, the more disappointed I was that sex education in the USA is so inadequate, but the better I was at having a compassionate understanding that bodies change, especially after reproductive trauma, changes in contraception, birth, and breastfeeding. And because my body changed, my sexual functioning changed too. It didn't mean I was less of a wife or woman, but it did give me some questions to ask about other things that could contribute. That is, was it lubrication that changed and then overall arousal, or was I less able to feel aroused in general? Had other areas of my sexual functioning diminished, like desire, orgasm, satisfaction, or pleasure? For me, the answers let me know it was a more comprehensive picture than just being wet or not.

All the things I described earlier, including the pandemic—which annihilated the introvert time I needed to feel like myself and cultivate sexual wanting, had negatively affected all but my capacity to orgasm. Writing this book, using the science I know, and practicing what I put into print has helped me as much as I hope it will be helpful to you. But it is a journey back, with just as many starts, stops, and hiccups as any other human has. The goal is not to be back to my old sexual self, as I thought it was before. It is to evolve in my sexuality and see the fruits of my career manifest in me and my sexual partner.

So, after a few relistens to "WAP" that fall, when I was striving to remember that joy had to be a part of the resistance, it kind of grew on me. Meg's first verse had a cadence that drew me in. The nostalgia took over, and of course I lived for the sisterhood the two rappers showed each other. I might have even stress tested my knees, trying to see if I could at least twerk right, since my days of doing splits and handstands are over. Dancing to "WAP" brought me a lot of joy, and I still use lube. I may never have WAP au naturel again, and I'm content with what my body can and cannot do.

16

Good Sex
is Safe

K im and Marcos met at twenty-six, when both were in graduate school in California. They were both conscientious about getting tested for STIs before they began exploring sexually. Marcos said, "The way I wanted to be able to give her pleasure, I didn't want anything to be off the table." So, when they got their test results back, he was happy to share, "Hey, my test says I'm clean and so are you!" Kim paused him.

"I've had an STI before, and I wasn't *dirty* then, so I'm not *clean* now. I'm just negative for any STIs. It is important for me to clarify that, because should either of our statuses change for whatever reason, I don't ever want to be shamed or shame you."

"Damn, I never even thought about it like that," he admitted. Marcos went on to explain that he took pride in never having had an STI, because in Puerto Rico, HIV was big for a while. "We were like in the top ten, so we had a bunch of sex education related to that. That was the language the teachers used. 'Clean bill of health.' But I do see how the opposite of that is dirty, and we definitely made people feel like that if we found out."

"Yeah, when I had to tell my ex that I tested positive for chlamydia, he said all kinds of rude shit, but he was the one that I contracted it from. He didn't want to get tested and confirm that though. It took a week to convince him, and when his results also came back positive, he finally apologized. I don't want to go through that again."

"My bad! I'm not judging you. I also hate that he tried to flip the script on you, rather than taking accountability."

DISCOMFORT V. DANGER

Safety is related to both preservation of health and protection from danger. It's also come to be associated with psychological safety, or a sense that one is not just kept from physical endangerment, but emotional and mental danger as well. Although psychological safety started off as a term used in industrial and occupational psychology, it's come to be used in many other spaces, including sexual health education. It's important to distinguish between safety and comfort. Sometimes, these two get mixed up in a way that can be harmful.

Feeling some discomfort is a normal part of growth. Just like exercise can make your body feel uncomfortable but is ultimately good for you, difficult conversations can also be uncomfortable. That doesn't necessarily mean they're unsafe. A safe conversation is one where there's no shaming, blaming, humiliation, or threats involved. Even in sex, experiencing discomfort is something you can talk through with your partner. However, a lack of safety goes beyond just feeling uncomfortable. If you feel unsafe, talking it out may not be enough. True safety requires action to address the threat, whether it's emotional manipulation in a sexual relationship or a hostile work environment.

TALKING IT OUT AND TAKING ACTION

Let's use condom use as an example of how safety involves both communication and action. Remember from the communication chapter that talking about condoms can be uncomfortable. People might have different ideas about what condoms mean. Some might think condoms mean you don't trust them, rather than seeing them as protection for both partners. Others might worry condoms make sex less enjoyable or spontaneous. Having open conversations about why you prefer condoms is important to clarify these assumptions.

However, talking isn't enough. Sometimes you need to take action to reinforce your boundary on condom use. Imagine you and your partner agreed on condoms for anal sex, but not vaginal or oral. If, during sex, your partner tries to move from vaginal to anal without a condom, stopping them might feel uncomfortable in the moment. But taking action, like saying "Hey, wait, condom for this" or putting your hand on their penis to pause things, is ultimately about safety. Your partner might feel frustrated with the pause, but whether they choose to respect your need for a condom becomes a question of consent and safety.

As discussed earlier, good sexual communication also involves talking about what happens if someone breaks a boundary. The kink community often excels in this area by setting clear "blueprints" for what happens if someone violates a previously agreed-upon limit. This could involve stopping sex entirely, using a safe word, or having a specific consequence discussed beforehand. Talking about these consequences up front helps ensure everyone feels safe and respected.

Some cultural recipes identify monogamy as the only safe sexual relationship option, but evidence suggests that sex is safe based on whether the people within the relationship (committed or not, monogamous or not) uphold the type of safety they've established in honest conversation. People in ostensibly monogamous relationships get STIs every day, and monogamy does not protect anyone from sexual violence. Monogamy can be as beautiful a relationship style as any, but when relationship and sexual scripts suggest that it is the ideal institution for sexual safety—in any definition of the word—it requires an understanding of where those myths came from. I'm saying this as a monogamously married person who chose that relationship type after consideration of many relationship types. At this season of our lives, monogamy works for us, but I'm not under the delusion that it affords me more protection or safety than if my husband and I had chosen any other relationship style. What keeps us healthy is our actions.

INTIMATE INJUSTICE AND SAFE SEX

People who have been diagnosed with STIs are as worthy of good sex as people who have not. That is a full and complete sentence. What makes this even a topic of discussion in this chapter is that most of us were taught to judge people who have contracted STIs with words like "dirty," "burnt," and "unclean" that stigmatize and dehumanize them. These words are evaluations of the morality, character, and overall worthiness of people who have STIs: an intimate injustice. Wanting to avoid contracting an STI and preserve your health makes sense, but stigmatizing people who have or have ever had STIs doesn't.

First, about 20 percent of the US population currently has an STI. STIs are common, albeit avoidable, and their prevalence differs based on racial groups and sexual identities. The intersection of racism, classism, heterosexism, Christianity, and ableism prop up inequities in health care, access to condoms and contraception, stigma, sexual stereotypes, and a host of other things that make mostly marginalized people rank at the top of the STI lists. Some science places blame squarely on individual decision-making and actions, but there are systems—and the scripts these systems produce—that contribute to the lack of safety many people feel sexually.

Second, when someone contracts other forms of communicable infection or disease, we're less likely to relate it to their morality than we are when it is sexual. My oldest son is in junior kindergarten. Kids have germs. I get the school sinus infection, and I am afforded sympathy. But if I kiss a romantic partner who has HSV and get a cold sore, I'd be more likely to be met with disgust and ridicule. No wonder people have such a difficult time with honest sexual communication related to disclosure of STI status. They fear being judged or humiliated, told that they're no longer worthy of good sex or even respect and care.

Safe sex is also about more than preventing STIs or unplanned pregnancies, although the subpar sex education most of us get would have us believe otherwise. Safe sex requires consent for it to even count as sex, rather than assault. The way we navigate consent in a power imbalanced society is ripe with cultural recipes about who can and cannot say no, or not this, or not now. Unfortunately, there are still people who think saying no to one's marital partner is sinful, rather than an expression of safe sex. So the rampancy of rape culture can make sex feel quite unsafe too.

PROTECTION FROM STIs AND UNWANTED PREGNANCY

Knowing the options for contraception can help you make informed choices about what type of protection works best for you and your sexual partner(s). Some types of contraception may require a conversation, and others may be exclusively your decision.

TYPES OF CONTRACEPTION

- **Hormonal Methods:** These methods use hormones to prevent pregnancy by suppressing ovulation (the release of an egg) or thickening cervical mucus to block sperm.
  - ▸ **Examples:** Birth control pills, implant, injection, patch, vaginal ring

- **Barrier Methods:** These methods create a physical barrier to prevent sperm from reaching the egg.
  - ▸ **Examples:** External condoms, internal condoms, spermicide (chemical foam/gel that kills sperm), cervical cap, diaphragm

- **Intrauterine Devices (IUDs):** A small, T-shaped device inserted into the uterus that prevents pregnancy for several years. IUDs work in different ways, depending on the type (hormonal and copper).

- **Fertility Awareness-Based Methods (FABMs):** These methods track the menstrual cycle to identify fertile windows (the days someone can get pregnant). You can then avoid sex during this time or use another form of contraception.
  - ▸ **Examples:** Calendar method, cervical mucus tracking, basal body temperature

- **Emergency Contraception (EC):** Also known as the "morning-after pill," EC is a high-dose hormone pill that can prevent pregnancy after unprotected sex. It's most effective the sooner you take it. The copper IUD can also be an EC.

- **Permanent Birth Control (Sterilization):** These methods are surgical procedures that block the fallopian tubes or vas deferens to permanently prevent pregnancy.
  - ▸ **Examples:** Tubal ligation, vasectomy (often reversable)

These contraceptive methods can be combined for increased protection. For example, an internal condom (also known as a female condom), can be used with an IUD to prevent STIs and unwanted pregnancy simultaneously. Barrier methods are the only contraceptives that can also prevent some STIs. But medicines like PrEP (pre-exposure prophylaxis), PEP (post-exposure prophylaxis), and Doxy-PEP (Doxycycline post-exposure prophylaxis) can prevent HIV (PrEP and PEP) and other STIs (Doxy-PEP) if you have non-barriered sex with someone with an STI.

SEXUAL VIOLENCE

Sexual violence is more common than most people realize, given that 50 percent of cis women and transgender people and 33 percent of cis men have experienced some form of sexual assault in their lifetime. The groups that face disproportionately high STI rates are often the same groups that are targeted for sexual violence. It may be because predators know they can get away with it without sanction or consequence most of the time. That said, the way to keep people safe from sexual violence is to prevent perpetrators from violating others. Outreach programs that increase knowledge about sexual violence in schools and communities are as necessary as programs that rehabilitate people who have already perpetrated, but the science is not yet clear on how effective these programs are. That means researchers need to do a better job of designing, implementing, and testing whether these programs reduce the rate of sexual violence perpetrated.

Unfortunately, the history of the USA is founded on the sexual violence and reproduction of Black and Indigenous people during enslavement and colonization. Frankly, we wouldn't have industrialized at the rate we did without them, so it wasn't just that white men got away with these atrocities without sanction. They were rewarded handsomely for the violence. When we talk about sexual safety as a modern concept, this history is omitted. Very few sex education classes, especially those taught in public schools, provide this essential context. Even in epidemiologists' surveys reporting the STI rates of marginalized groups, they are often reported ahistorically and decontextualized. Studies show that men who sleep with men, whether they identify as gay, bisexual, or not, face the highest rates of STIs, and only recently have those studies evaluated the extent to which systemic heterosexism contributes to their lack of safety and deaths.

So yes, we do need to show people how to use condoms, contraceptives, and to plan for and discuss options for sexual safety. But we should also be prepared with the ability to have nuanced conversations about all of this.

STRATEGIES FOR SAFE SEX

First, when you consider your safety needs, consider them alongside your positionality—all the privileged and marginalized identities you hold, as well as the histories (personal and generational) that influence your meaning making about who you are. For Kim, who comes from a culture that has relatively low STI rates in the USA, contracting an STI from her ex-partner brought up internalized stigma as well as concern for her health. When he responded defensively by shaming her, it capitalized on the stigma she was already feeling, but she also had courage to continue the conversation until he, too, got tested and learned his STI status. Through that lesson, she had to evaluate why she thought she was a bad person for contracting an STI (moralism, ableism), what made it hard for her to set condom use boundaries with her ex (sexism), and what type of sexual partner and dynamic she would prefer for her next relationship.

By the time she and Marcos met, she was clearer on that, evidenced by her ability to tell him "clean" wasn't a word she would use to describe her sexual health status. For Marcos, who comes from a culture that has a relatively high HIV rate, albeit lower rates for other STIs, the colonial mindset coupled with ableism in a way that socialized him to perpetuate unintentional sexual shaming of people who have STIs. The caring, but assertive, correction from Kim opened his eyes to see how hurtful that could be, and he opted to be more compassionate. These considerations may require reading or listening to resources that tell you more about your heritage and history as it relates to sex. You can also look to the CDC to see what the STI rates are in your city if you're dating, to know what the actual level of risk may be.

Second, you can make safe sex fun, but the resources you have access to make a difference: this is also related to intimate justice. Do you have access to a health care provider you trust and can share sexual health concerns with? Do you have access to all the types of contraception presented earlier in this chapter? If not, seeking out a health provider can include interviewing people to find the one that feels right for you. This should be someone who will gladly explore all contraceptive options you're interested in, rather than forcing some over others based on their prejudices.

Also, if you're having sex with someone you've agreed to use contraceptives with, try on a variety of condoms and barriers like dental dams, including internal and external. I'm partial to the internal condoms for the room they provide and the flexibility on when you can insert them. Practice various ways to communicate consent. The way we're taught about safe sex can have an element of play and joy to it. Sex educators are bringing in music, condom competitions, Q+A sessions, and sexy names. On the other hand, if you got the "don't be a boy's garbage can" public high school sex education like I did, you'll have to go looking for the more interesting, comprehensive versions of sex ed. I'm a sex therapist and a sex researcher, not a sex educator, so the 10 BIPOC Sex Educators You Need to Know list by LoversStores.com provides you with outstanding options of people to learn even more from.

17

Good Sex
is Relaxing

Insomnia had troubled Sincere on and off for decades. During adolescence, her mother asked her if the ancestors visited her at night and made it difficult for her to rest. Sincere didn't recall having spiritual guests, she told her mother. It felt more like her thoughts and ideas were most vibrant once she lay down to rest. Some of the thoughts were more like worries, but others were more creative. During summers, when she didn't have school, the insomnia allowed her to create beautiful, inspired oil paintings and pottery. During the school year, and now on workdays, she only allowed insomnia to inspire her on the weekends. For the weekdays, or when she had something important to do in the morning, she used masturbation to alleviate the stress and help her relax enough to fall asleep.

Her sleep routine was now a beautiful ritual in her elder years. Around ten o'clock in the evening, she ensured all sounds except nature were inaudible. She dabbed lavender essential oil directly on her pillow, just under the pillowcase. She eliminated as much light as possible with closed blackout curtains and a dual-purpose sleeping mask made of terry cloth to absorb some of the menopause-induced night sweats and block any remaining light. Then she thanked her ancestors for the day, especially any notably beautiful or hard things she experienced. She expressed gratitude while breathing in deep nasal inhales with long, open-mouthed sigh exhales, while she touched her inner thighs, then her vulva, then her clitoris.

Typically, she fell asleep soon after orgasm and remained asleep through the night, but occasionally just the genital touch and deep breathing were enough to relax her into slumber. As a community sex educator, she shared this tip with anyone who noted their fatigue and sleeplessness as a starting point. Even though Sincere had never felt, nor wanted to feel, sexual desire, her best medicine for a few tension and stress-related ailments was solo sex.

WHY WE NEED TO RELAX

An early definition of *relax* beautifully captures something many people are missing in a fast-paced, capitalist world: "set free, soften, reduce." So, related to liberation, getting the tension out of one's body and reducing the load of stress, relaxing sex can be an intervention for intimate justice.

As noted in the chapter on sensuality, most people are moving faster than serves them just to keep up with the everyday demands of life. We're not even talking about extracurriculars, just survival. Some of my research examines racial trauma and race-based stress, which is the "enduring cognitive, affective, and/or somatic responses to racism, including race-based stress reactions and subsequent race-based stress symptoms, that may manifest based on the intensity and/or frequency of racist stressors a person has experienced or witnessed." People with other marginalized identities, like women, trans people, queer people, older people, fat people, etc. also experience related minority or marginalization stress. Since most of us have multiple marginalized identities, intersectional stress and trauma are the reality. That is why it is essential that we make relaxation, sexual or otherwise, a part of our health and wellness praxis.

RELAXATION AS A SEXUAL HEALTH BENEFIT

The health benefits to good sex are plentiful, including reducing cramps, helping the prostate, and improving cardiovascular health. But one of the most well-known benefits is the relaxation that follows a good sex session. Many people use solo and partnered sex for stress and tension relief, because it can work better than massage and even some medicines. It's organic and orgasmic. Carolyn Meiller and I studied masturbation among queer women, and some suggested it provided stress reduction and release. In fact, a common reason people masturbate outside of pleasure and enjoyment is to fall asleep. If you've ever had a post-nut slumber, you know how true this is.

Additionally, research points to the employment of sex workers, especially during sex tourism, as related to a desire for relaxation. Chris Ryan and Rachel Kinder suggest that the same reasons people take vacations are reflected in the reasons people opt to engage sex workers: relaxation. Sex workers can and do provide many services that are within and outside of mainstream cultural recipes for what sex should be because they already knowingly occupy a position of marginality, not just in their occupation, but often along the lines of their socioeconomic status (current or of origin), race, and attitudes about what sex is and isn't. Some people engaged in sex work, like those engaged in other less stigmatized care-based professions, see their work as helping people to relax and enjoy pleasure. Others see it to a financial end. Many see it as both. But, understanding the different types of sex workers and the social sanctions they face in many places, it makes sense to assume their services are valuable in stress reduction and relaxation because it is an old profession that stands despite legality.

Most people living in the USA reported moderate levels of stress in 2022, a five out of ten, but these levels are higher than the pre-pandemic era. Finances, sociopolitical climate, family, and work are some of the stressors people navigate daily. Over one-quarter of adults say the stress is so bad they cannot function most of the time. That amount of distress has negative health consequences, including low quality of life and early death, but many people underestimate the value of good sex as one of many free strategies available to reduce stress. With so many sex-negative messages about being sexual, despite the normalcy of sex, people come to believe it's pathological to enjoy sex as a form of relaxation. But relaxation, or stress reduction, remains one of the most reported reasons people have sex.

For some people, however, sexual anxiety can get in the way of realizing the relaxation of good sex. Sexual anxiety includes feelings of worry or fear associated with initiating or participating in a sexual experience. Some people experience it as a function of generalized anxiety disorder—basically they are anxious about most things and sex is not exempt. Other people have situational anxieties that mostly include sex. So the worry creeps in when they feel they must perform a certain way, look just so, or be receptive to sex despite discomfort or pain they may feel. Sexual anxiety can be a precursor to genito-pelvic pain disorders. These disorders are typically the physiological contraction of the vaginal opening or pelvic floor, such that penetration is incredibly painful to impossible. But many people don't realize that oral and nonpenetrative manual sex are options for sex that don't require vaginismus and other genito-pelvic pain disorders to completely subside. Some people make penetration the goal, rather than having a good sexual experience, which in turn results in heightened sexual anxiety due to fear it won't work well.

Sexually anxious people with penises may struggle with maintaining an erection or they may ejaculate faster than intended. Again, with performance anxieties common among men who believe their value is in their sexual prowess, sexual dysfunction can be experienced with shame. It's incredibly hard to relax when you feel ashamed that you're not as erect as you or your partner want you to be. So even if an erection eventually arises, it may not last long. Remember that there are other ways people with penises can enjoy sex without penetrating or having an erection. And, premature ejaculation may not be as bad as they think. Prostate massage is one example of a way to provide an unerect sexual partner stimulation and maybe even ejaculation without penetration.

WHICH SEX IS MOST RELAXING

The research doesn't provide clear answers on whether solo sex is more relaxing than partnered sex, because it depends on the positionality of the person(s) having sex. It's probably easier to use solo sex for relaxation because there isn't the added desire for reciprocity. If you are experiencing stress, and you just want to relax, it's less likely that you have the energy or desire to do what it takes to address your partner's sexual desires at that time, whatever they may be. It's also harder to tell someone that you're not paying that you only want to feel relaxed and not engage in a mutually relaxing experience, even if it's true. But there are occasions where both partners have had a day. Both want to relax, and sex is a way to help them feel reconnected with each other, which in turn allows for the relaxation.

On the other hand, solo sex can be helpfully selfish. You only have to attend to your own sexual experience, and the position, pace, and purpose of the sexual experience are tailored to what you need. If it is relaxation, and you just want to lie there like a log while the vibrator shakes the stress off you, there's no nagging feeling in the back of your mind that you are letting your partner down. You're just trying to get to a more relaxed state, and it works.

STRATEGIES FOR RELAXATION: SEX TO SLEEP

How much do you need relaxation right now? Track your stress levels for a week prior to trying any of these strategies to get a baseline for how stressed, tense, or overwhelmed you've been feeling overall. You can simply use a number from zero—no stress at all—to ten—the most stressed I've ever felt—and write it in a notebook or notes app on your phone at the end of each day.

For solo sex, you can follow a process like Sincere. At a dedicated bedtime, make sure to avoid phones and other screens for an hour before you want to fall asleep. If possible, remove all sounds except for nature or relaxing, lyricless music. Choose an essential oil that helps with relaxation and dab it under your pillowcase. Use dim, soft lighting or darkness. Take deep breaths in through your nose and out through your mouth as you express gratitude for the day. Then, touch your body, including genitals, gently at first. Then, use whatever technique works best for your relaxation.

For partnered sex, co-regulation techniques can help make sex a relaxing experience. Try activities like matched breathing, eye gazing, and deep cuddling before, during, or after the sexual experience. For example, synchronizing your breathing while looking into each other's eyes after a sexual experience can help both partners relax and relieve stress. Breathing in for five seconds and out for seven in concert for a few minutes, holding each other close, and looking into each other's eyes can help your nervous systems calm down. Keep towels, or other things you may use to wipe up as needed, warm and next to the place you're having sex, so neither one of you has to get up. Or just lie in it and fall asleep sticky. Prioritize sleep over the clean up.

For Sincere, who was not in conflict with her sleeping style during nonwork times, the use of solo sex for her relaxation was a healthy option. Sleep is such a cornerstone of good health, and good sex is one underutilized option to increase the likelihood that you get relaxed enough to enjoy the sleep you need. The Nap Bishop Tricia Hersey says, "rest is resistance," because many of us have not been afforded adequate rest historically and currently. I say relaxation is resistance too, whether it is sleep or not.

Whether people experience pleasure and desire for sex or not, such as people who identify as asexual, the use of sex to relax is a benefit anyone can receive. It would be interesting to see if any studies compare sex with other sleep or relaxation aids to determine which one is most effective, but it is always useful to have many options to reduce stress and increase relaxation, rather than just one upon which we over rely. So, if you don't already have it on the list, add sex to your relaxation repertoire.

18

Good Sex
is Comfortable

n almost every sense of the word, Tim had lived a life of comfort. Offering privilege in nearly all aspects of his identity, the systems worked overtime extracting comfort from others to ensure his comfort as a white, middle-class, able-bodied, educated, heterosexual cis man was an expected experience. If he walked into a room where there were people that didn't share his identities, most of them would consciously or subconsciously shift themselves in language, disposition, and otherwise to maintain his comfort. It was something so normal to him that he took it for granted. He often felt entitled to comfort without realizing he was acting from an entitled place, as we came to explore therapeutically.

He expected people would smile at him and offer him the best customer service when he walked into a store to purchase what he wanted. He expected that if he just worked hard enough, he would achieve all the goals he set for himself. He expected that there would be ease, minimal pain that he didn't self-inflict, and care when pain or even temporary discomfort came to him. He got to experience what most of us are worthy of his entire life. Having a Black woman as a therapist offered him the gift of an honest mirror, especially as he began exploring his emerging identity as someone who enjoyed cross-dressing and other kinks.

Where I could hold compassion for his heartbreak when his wife left him, the visceral pain that the woman he loved may not accept him for who he was discovering himself to be, I also could offer that he hadn't developed the capacity to hold her point of view. He didn't have to agree with her viewpoint, but the process of holding it and sitting with discomfort could teach him something valuable about her willingness to share it. When he began to express the expansiveness of his gender, it was clear that he hadn't been presented with the opportunity to develop resilience on his own yet. His stoic shutdown was a response to his overwhelm with what it might mean to be on a margin. And so, when it came to his sex life, where comfort was a byproduct of his privilege, rather than any work he had to do to create comfort for himself, he had to learn to be better balanced in offering comfort, rather than receiving it.

SOOTHING AND EASING PAIN

Comfort can be lovely, but discomfort isn't always a bad thing, as discussed in the safe chapter. Early definitions of *comfort* dating back to the 1300s include "consoling and soothing, especially from grief or trouble." It also includes references to fortifying and strengthening the person needing comfort. More modern definitions refer to physical ease. Experiencing comfort in the context of sex, then, recognizes the need for potential adjustments on behalf of both partners to afford each other ease, soothing, and strengthening. The absence of physical pain is also important to sexual comfort. Does your body have the capacity to experience certain components of sex and not others? Nothing wrong with that. But do you continue to engage in the types of sex that your body cannot experience without pain because they are the most familiar activities or the ones preferred by your partner? In that case, it's likely you have lower sexual comfort.

In the previous chapter, I referenced genito-pelvic pain disorders that emerge due to sexual anxiety. However, there are pain disorders that come before or without any associated anxiety or tension too. Vulvodynia is one where the vaginal glands, rather than an unrelaxed vaginal wall, make having sex painful. Although anxiety and fear may arise after the sex has been painful a few times, over time, the reason the pain began has nothing to do with lack of relaxation or high anxiety. Providing sexual comfort, or learning ways to help avoid, reduce, or eliminate pain, to someone who experiences this sexual dysfunction is one way to participate in good sex.

There are also aspects of one's physical ability status and age status that can create discomfort and pain. Lack of mobility or flexibility, for instance, can make certain positions nearly unbearable. And just because you were able to do a position at one point in your life doesn't mean you should always be able to do it. Bodies change. Capacities change. High school cheer captain me and forty-one-year-old mom me have drastically different levels of flexibility. I could work overtime to try to regain some of it, but it's likely that it all ain't coming back. As another example, people with physical disabilities have some beautiful ways of approaching sex with assistive technology like chairs, pillows, and supports that facilitate sexual comfort, but without them their bodies may not be able to experience certain types of sex enjoyably.

Ableist cultural recipes that make us think sex must be a certain way, with certain positions, for a certain length of time, etc. serve as barriers to sexual comfort. Having a sexual partner that gets you, really appreciates the fullness of your humanity, on the other hand, can be a great disruption to these harmful sexual scripts. Sex partners that take consideration to avoid causing pain and to accommodate potentially ever-changing needs of ever-changing bodies are hallmarks of good sex. Older adults who have maintained healthy, good sex lives can be valuable sources of wisdom. Unfortunately, stereotypes about sex being for the young and societal taboos against older adults discussing sex can prevent this knowledge from being shared. By openly talking about sex across generations, we can create a culture of good sex for everyone.

FEELING NATURAL, NOT PAINFUL

In Breanne Fahs and Rebecca Plante's paper about cis women's definitions of good, happy, and joyous sex, comfort emerged as one of the themes. While the previous chapter on relaxation and sex indicated it can be experienced within nearly any sexual encounter, comfort appears to have a time-based element according to their research. Longevity in the relationship seemed to lead to greater intimacy, which in turn contributed to greater sexual comfort. Their participants describe it as feeling ease or feeling "natural" with a sexual partner. That is, the sexual experience doesn't feel contrived or forced, they're just going with the flow.

Studies by Jardin Dogan, Shemeka Thorpe, and Natalie Malone have explored how Black cis women cope with sexual pain. They found that the pressure to embody the "strong Black woman" stereotype discouraged the women from seeking help. They worried their partners would see them as weak if they admitted to experiencing pain. This often led them to suffer in silence, even avoiding discussing it with health care providers. Unfortunately, some who did speak to health care providers felt dismissed or unheard.

These findings suggest a two-pronged approach is needed to address sexual pain in Black women. First, we need to develop new ways to talk about sexual pain within relationships. This could involve finding language that empowers Black women to express their needs without feeling judged. Second, health care systems need to improve how they address sexual pain concerns, particularly from Black women. This might involve cultural sensitivity training for doctors and creating a more supportive environment for open communication about sexual health. More research is needed to represent how this shows up for women with other racially marginalized identities, but, in many ways, these recommendations can work for people regardless of identity. This would support the erotic equity we need.

New research can also examine how sexual partners with multiple privileged identities can learn to be an avenue of sexual comfort to their partners, especially when their partners are more marginalized than they are. For example, what would someone like Tim need to learn to make it feel natural or comfortable for him and his wife?

STRATEGIES FOR SEXUAL COMFORT

There are several questions you need to answer that inform you about your relationship to sexual comfort. If you are partnered, it may be helpful to discuss them together, so you're each better prepared to facilitate comfort and receive it.

- What are the things that make sex comfortable for you?

- Do other parts of sex feel enriched when you are comfortable with your sexual partner(s)?

- If your sexual partner is experiencing discomfort or pain, is it something you notice without their verbal communication, or do they need to tell you more directly?

- Do you feel like you share responsibility for the comfort in your sexual relationships, or is it only your responsibility to address your own comfort, while your partner addresses theirs?

- In what other areas of your life are you used to comfort?

- In what areas of your life is comfort more of a luxury than the standard?

- Do you have any negative messages sitting with you about who deserves and does not deserve comfort?

- Within these messages, where do you place your own worthiness?

- Do you work to make others comfortable at the expense of your own, sexually or nonsexually?

These questions are designed to guide you to examine your relationship with comfort in general and sexually. Tim and I found that when he was able to discuss his orientation to comfort honestly, he assumed other people were receiving the comfort-inducing benefits he received as a hetero white man in the world. When they weren't, he believed they must have done something to disrupt the always available comforts, rather than seeing himself as the beneficiary of most people's care and comforting energy.

One activity we used was for him to go into grocery stores in different neighborhoods, those that were and were not predominantly white, and notice how the cashier addressed him versus the person before him or after him. He expected that he would receive good customer service in the white stores but not in the stores with predominantly people of the global majority. He was correct on the first account and wrong on the second. In both stores, regardless of how other patrons were treated, he was treated well.

Then I had him reflect on his sexual experiences, including those predating his relationship with his wife. He recalled, somewhat embarrassed, that he assumed his partners were as comfortable asking for what they wanted as he was. He assumed they were comfortable with their bodies just because he found them attractive. He called one with whom he remained friends to ask her about whether she always experienced comfort with him. Just noticing the hesitation of her answer was an answer. When she finally spoke, she named the many ways she had sexually accommodated him to ensure his comfort with hopes that it would make her seem like an ideal girlfriend and potential wife. "I never really was myself around you," she admitted.

Once he and his wife decided to try again, we had a couple's session to discuss comfort, where she expressed that a part of her leaving was to prioritize her comfort over his. "I could have acquiesced easier, but frankly I was tired of you thinking you deserved it automatically. I needed the time I needed to see how I could . . . if I could . . . return to our marriage and experience you sexually knowing about your gender stuff."

He admitted, "I would not have been able to seek out the type of kink I needed to help me process this comfort paradigm if you didn't leave. For that I am grateful. I also better understand now what my comfort has cost you and other people I have cared about, inside and outside of the bedroom."

After answering the questions above, each partner in the sexual relationship should take one week to be the focus of comfort. You can choose whether this is exclusive to sexual comfort or comfort throughout the relationship. That means, for one week, all people will only prioritize one person's comfort and focus on the things that make them most comfortable. At the end of the experience, check in with how shifting the dynamic around comfort reveals any erotic inequities. This is what Tim and his wife did.

The repair work they both agreed to in their relationship was a six-month trial of her comfort being prioritized sexually and relationally, no matter what. It was difficult for both of them to occupy the new roles, but it was useful in calculating the cost of focusing on the comfort of a single person rather than holding a reciprocal sexual comfort frame. She asked for things she would have held her tongue about earlier, including small things like a pillow for her lower back during oral sex. Before this exercise, she would have just sucked it up and assumed she should be grateful he was interested in giving oral. Just a simple change in angle and support helped her alignment and experience of that pleasure. At the end of the six months, long enough where it couldn't be faked, they were able to approach their sex life and marriage with more balance, ease, and shared growth-oriented discomfort that would not dissipate completely for anyone who wanted to maintain the healthy balance.

— 19 —

Good Sex
is Liberating

In their daily lives, Nakita and Joi were activists. They'd been doing frontline work in their community for the Movement for Black Lives since 2013 individually, and they met through the community garden Nakita launched. Social justice work was not new to them, so they were surprised to find that intimate justice was an area that could use some exploration. Because liberation in many forms was important, they were willing to go there to explore what sexual liberation could be for them.

"I thought I was so much further along in my liberation journey, then I met Nakita. She seemed so much further along than I did, because I didn't even realize some of the things in my life that were shaping me . . . things like my hair texture," said Joi.

"Yeah, she was wearing a Dominican blowout when we met, and there's nothing wrong with that. But when she felt embarrassed to let me see her without her hair straight, scared to make love to me in the shower because her hair would show up as its normal self, I asked her what she was afraid of." Nakita touched Joi's curls, proud to see her partner's texture outside of the house.

"Finding out I'm afraid of my Blackness, while dating a Black woman was wild." Joi shook her head in embarrassment.

"I think because I present more masculine of center, and I'm dark skinned and fat with a short cut, she didn't realize I had to go through years of people considering me ugly because I didn't look like her. It was kids doing and saying kid shit, hurtful for sure, but I got really grounded in myself and who I was through that time."

"In my family, 'pretty' had a certain look, and I came very close except for my hair. Keeping it straight helped me stay safe, or at least it felt that way, safe from all the stuff she was probably going through. So when she asked me why I wouldn't do shower sex, I realized I was afraid of losing that privilege, the vulnerability of not reflecting this ideal. Would I still be desirable to her if my hair wasn't straight?"

"Which is hilarious because I couldn't give less of a fuck about her hair texture. I know damn well her hair isn't naturally straight. I was trying to get ate out in the shower."

We laughed until we cried, all three of us. Working with Nakita on sexual fun and excitement, our therapeutic relationship had a lot of joyful moments to bolster the impact of the deep work. Now we were getting to inner child and family systems, which is often the first direct imprint on our sexual selves. Families translate the cultural recipes to us from the ingredients they were given unless they were allowed to revise the recipes. Most weren't allowed, nor were they given access to better ingredients for good sex. That is intimate injustice, and sexual liberation is a totally new menu.

SETTING YOUR SEXUAL SELF FREE

Liberation is an older concept than the word indicates. The etymology of the word suggests it emerged in the 1500s to mean "setting free from restraint or confinement." Sydelle Barreto defines *sexual libera-tion* as the "unimpeded, authentic construction of our sexual selves." Taken together, it means getting set free to develop an authentic sexual self. Most of us have a variety of "isms" from which we need to be liberated, and there are very few of us who have absolutely nothing that has us shackled. So sexual liberation is a type of resistance that has been an evergreen part of the human sexual experience across cultures and time.

Breanne Fahs refers to this as "freedom from" sexual liberation, which must be coupled with "freedom to" sexual liberation to really meet the mark. The former contextualizes what intersectional oppressions prevent us from enjoying our holistic, authentic sexual selves. The latter permits us to explore a variety of consensual sexual experiences that help shape who our authentic, liberated sexual selves are. Each ingredient in this book is an option on the sexual liberation menu.

According to Barreto, who discusses sexual liberation in the context of fat liberation, "the process of sexual self-making [. . .] can also be a way of understanding sexual liberation." Also known as sexual subjectivity, sexual self-making is core to sexual liberation, and it happens in a context of privilege and marginalization. A privilege portfolio exercise might help you better understand in what areas you are doing the shackling (inadvertently or actively) and what areas you might need liberation. This will come later in this chapter. But for now, consider the function of liberation.

My maternal grandmother, who I lived with on and off until I was twelve, is a Jehovah's Witness. I'm not. In our small town in Western New York, you knew the kids who were because they didn't attend birthday parties, didn't celebrate any holidays, and they didn't say the Pledge of Allegiance. They weren't indoctrinated, like the rest of us, with the daily recitation of "I pledge allegiance, to the flag . . ." My public-school attendees know the rest.

I don't say the pledge or sing the national anthem anymore, even though I used to love patriotic songs. But I still rock with "liberty and justice for all" as a solid aspiration for the USA. It resonates deeply with me, and if "liberty and justice for all" is a supposed American value, then liberation is the process to get there. People who are working toward liberation recognize that we've not fully actualized the value of liberty, here or anywhere in the world. As I write this book, conservative agents are banning books like this from libraries and schools. Liberation remains aspirational, but we're often not taught the skills to get there. People laugh when I suggest that our sex lives are a primary site of liberation, a place where we can get free. Because sex is typically private or intimate, some people feel like sexual liberation isn't big enough to qualify for a movement. It seems to only affect the individuals involved. Intimate justice frames this differently.

Intimate justice, as I've discussed earlier, reflects that the private relationship and the functions of them (care, sex, and other intimate labors and offerings) are a ripe practice ground for any liberation movement: how you act in your bedroom, how you parent, how you engage your siblings, how you treat your lovers and reflect on your use of power to liberate or dominate, both yourself and them.

We all have power, even when it feels like we don't, but most of our social systems wouldn't have us believe that. It doesn't serve oppression when you realize your power and are willing to risk some of the trappings of privilege to use your power in service of liberation. Good sex is an opportunity to do just that.

Forced or unexamined inhibitions are one of the ways oppressions can play out in our sex lives. We internalize the unseasoned sexual menu and cultural recipes that tell us who is deserving of good sex and what good sex should be early in life, then we get a set of limited ingredients. Often unknowingly, we restrict ourselves and our behaviors to try to fit those recipes, missing out on the deliciousness available to us. Now, some of us are rebellious to the core, natural resisters, and disruptors. But most people, if you're being honest, do not feel capable of tolerating the isolation and abandonment at stake with liberation. And depending on how much intersecting marginalization you're contending with, the threats to your life are so numerous that it makes sense when you shrink to survive.

THREE LEVELS OF RISK

There are three levels of risk we all must consider when opting for liberation: life risks, livelihood risks, and luxury risks. Some of us experience life risks, meaning you could be killed or harmed for pursuing liberation. We know many people by name who have been assassinated or lost their lives due to liberation efforts, such as Malcolm X (racial rights leader) and Marsha P. Johnson (trans rights leader).

Then there are more of us who experience livelihood risks, meaning the ability to provide resources for yourself or the people within your care is compromised or extinguished based on your commitment to liberation. For example, people have lost their jobs or been ostracized for even mentioning racism, sexism, or heterosexism at work. As I write this, University of Florida staff with diversity, equity, and inclusion roles were terminated from their jobs. Participants in labor union protests have had to give up pay to advocate for decent wages.

Last, nearly all of us have to risk luxuries to realize liberation. I don't know a single person who has undertaken a liberation journey and lost nothing. Luxury risks include the risk of isolation, less access to privileges, or having your reputation maligned. Don't get me wrong, these things feel terrible, but they are not the same as livelihood or life risks, even if our bodies and emotions make it feel that way.

Frankly, some of us are at risk of losing the luxury of romantic partnership with certain people if we attempt to journey toward liberation in our sexual relationships. It can feel scary to even ask for what you want from a partner, for example wanting to use condoms, because you fear they may reject you. But good sex, sex that is good *to* and good *for* everyone involved, is designed to facilitate liberation.

Sherronda J. Brown, author of *Refusing Compulsory Sexuality: A Black Asexual Lens on Our Sex-Obsessed Culture*, says, "What I have come to learn after many years of studying, thinking, and writing about power and oppression is that there will always be factions of marginalized people who do not want collective liberation from the oppressive systems we live and die under. Liberation is simply too big, too daunting, too difficult to fathom. What these people resort to instead is the creation and maintenance of systems in which they can act as oppressors and wield what little power they do have over others. If the world must be structured through hierarchies, then marginalized people who are not fully committed to liberation, or the dismantling of these hierarchies, must find a way to never be at the bottom." Welp.

I mean, Sherronda said what needed to be said, and many of us have observed this in action, but it still feels upsetting and painful to witness it. To me, it suggests a lack of capacity for radical imagination, hope, and commitment to action, but it also reflects a deeply rooted sense of hopelessness. It's unfortunately a symptom of oppression that keeps the system working, and on occasion we don't even realize how we're complicit in this. Dedicating or withholding the energy and patience it takes to contribute to an orgasmic experience for your partner after you've already come is a sex example. It seems small, but this decision reinforces a power differential that suggests one partner's orgasm is more important than the other's.

SELF-DEFINING SEXUAL LIBERATION

Young Black women defining sexual liberation for themselves is relevant for so many groups because of the intersecting oppression (racism and sexism, at least) they're facing. Jeannette Wade and colleagues led several focus groups where they found young Black women suggested sexual liberation included ownership, awareness, confidence, and pleasure.

- Ownership includes autonomy in your sexual decision-making, free from unwanted social pressure on those decisions.

- Awareness related to knowing what you do and do not want sexually. I'd add that what you're being liberated from should be included in your sexual self-awareness.

- Confidence included how those aspects of knowing are communicated with sexual partners. Being unapologetic and trusting yourself were hallmarks of confidence too.

- Pleasure—an aspect of good sex already described in Chapter 3—was defined by the women in their study as physical and emotional enjoyment.

Intimate justice recognizes that not everyone has equal and fair access to these components of sexual liberation. For example, awareness is limited by lack of comprehensive sex education in most schools. This systemic issue is likely driven by capitalism, heterosexism, and purity culture—at a minimum. Similarly, the systemic racism that begets texturism (privileging of straight hair over other textures) prevented Joi from embracing her authentic sexual self and realizing sexual liberation too. It was easy for her to overlook it because her awareness was compromised by growing up in Dominican culture, where the texturism is normalized in good hair/bad hair discourse. This typically happens in intimate relationships with family members, peers, and partners.

My team's research explored how people experience power in sex. We looked at how people describe their first and most recent sexual encounters, focusing on a range of feelings—from powerless to empowered. We found that feeling like they had control over their sexual choices (sexual autonomy) was linked to feeling empowered during sex. This aligns with the idea of "ownership" put forth by Wade.

Stories of sexual empowerment often included descriptions of pleasure, feeling in control (agency), and joy. These elements combined paint a picture of sexual liberation. Interestingly, for Black people of all genders, simply being able to talk openly about vulnerability and negative emotions during sex was also seen as a form of liberation. This challenges stereotypes like "strong Black woman" and "John Henryism," which portray Black people as incapable of feeling vulnerable. Therefore, the ability to discuss sexual experiences across the power spectrum itself becomes an act of sexual liberation.

What we need to get free from to enjoy sexual liberation may be something that directly or indirectly impacts good sex. For example, internalized texturism was directly impacting good sex for Joi, whereas systemic and interpersonal racism may have indirectly impacted good sex for Nakita. Additionally, participating in your own liberation and the liberation of anyone you have sex with requires developing awareness of your power and how you use it.

STRATEGIES FOR SEXUAL LIBERATION

First, to develop awareness of the areas where you are privileged, create your privilege portfolio. In the list below, circle your current identities, recognizing that some of the identities can change over time.

- White
- Male
- Cis
- Middle class or higher
- Tall
- Able-bodied
- Heterosexual
- Ages twenty-two to fifty-five

- Christian
- Stereotypically attractive
- College-educated
- Neurotypical
- English-speaking
- Citizen of the USA
- Slim-bodied

Once you've circled all your privileged identities, count them. When I'm leading workshops, the typical range of privileged identities among participants is nine to fourteen. I have eleven at this moment in time. Understanding this helps increase awareness about the amount of power that is bestowed upon you, whether earned or unearned, felt or unfelt.

Next, ask yourself, "In what way do I use my power to dominate, rather than liberate, in sex?" The self-work is essential before you go to the next question, which is, "In what ways does my partner(s) use their power to dominate, rather than liberate, me sexually?" Some of the examples I've heard include withholding sex to win an argument, guilting someone into or out of different types of sex, shaming someone for their consensual sexual choices, and being sexually self-centered rather than reciprocal. If we're honest, most of us are going to be able to answer both questions. Most of us, regardless of how little privilege in your portfolio, will have examples of ways we've participated in the subjugation of other people, but hopefully we're also able to answer the question affirmatively about being able to contribute to a partner's liberation.

I regret shaming a former partner for his penis size when the condom came off unintentionally. Rather than maturely addressing our options at that point, twenty-one-year-old me lashed out and never spoke to him again. In that instance, I allowed my fear about being impregnated before I was ready—by someone I didn't want a long-term future with—turn into a verbal attack. That is using my power to oppress. If you ever read this and know who you are, I sincerely apologize for my behavior. You didn't deserve that.

What you may come to learn is that liberation is about releasing the desire to control or the entitlement to feel as if you get to control others, just because they're involved with you in some way. At best, we can make invitations and set boundaries with honest intention that allow others to consent into the sexual experience we're hoping to have. But control is a hallmark of oppressive domination, and it's often born from anxieties and insecurities. We don't need to control others when we feel inherently secure and worthy ourselves.

Next, ask yourself, "In what ways do I use my power to liberate myself and my partner in sex? In what ways does my partner(s) use their power to liberate me?" Recalling stories of a time when someone you had sex with promoted your sexual empowerment and liberation, by building your awareness, confidence, ownership, or pleasure, and when you did the same for someone else can help you identify what actions were most freeing.

Another question to consider is, "When have I been most likely to act oppressively in sexual relationships with myself and others?" Really consider what you felt during those times and what cultural recipes you drew on to justify the controlling actions. Provide as many contextual details as you can remember. Finally, "When have I been most likely to act in liberating ways in my sexual relationships with myself and others?" Consider the same things you considered above. This will help you parse out what needs you were trying to fulfill, where the ideas came from, and what contexts supported domination or liberation, so you can lean into or away from them.

With these questions answered, you have clarified the boundaries of your sexual liberation window. In your next sexual experience, choose to add at least one liberation facilitator and remove one liberation barrier. You can talk about what these might be with your partner beforehand. For example, if you realize asking your partner to use a condom was much easier when you didn't fear abandonment, you can talk with them about an experience where you felt more powerless in condom negotiation before and what would help you feel empowered next time.

SEX AS A SITE OF LIBERATION

So, what can sex liberate us from? All the isms. In meaningful ways. Returning to Nakita and Joi, at first, I had Joi share a picture with Nakita of her as a child with curly hair. I had Nakita share a childhood picture with Joi too. I had them both choose the picture they thought was the most cringe, because the vulnerability we were working up to in their sex lives was going to require inner child work first. I had them each tell a story about what those little girls knew, felt, dreamed, and wanted in life. What did those little girls need to hear to assure them that they were inherently worthy as is, no changes needed?

Through tears from both women, we processed the ways colorism, texturism, sexism, heterosexism, and racism had tried to bind them to specific ways of knowing themselves that they often had reinforced in close relationships. Then I assigned homework where both write messages to both little girls, the girls they were, and the girls their partners used to be. Once they read those letters to each other, they washed each other's hair while using affirmations to counteract damaging messages each had received. They then made love with their hair in its washed, natural state. In the next session, Nakita shared that she did, indeed, get to enjoy head in the shower.

CONCLUSION

This book is presented more like a menu than a manual. There are many good sex ingredients outlined that may not resonate for your specific menu of good sex. If good sex is pleasurable, orgasmic, and intimate for you, you have likely read the stories, sexual scripts, science, and strategies that relate to those menu items laid out in each chapter. It's also important to remember the human you are reading this book, and the human I am writing it, because our shared and different identities make up the way we'll be able to use the information in this book.

I wrote this book while pregnant with, and then nursing, my second child, but it was my third pregnancy. The first and third pregnancies were as overall good as a pregnancy could ever be. The second nearly ended my life. So, as I wrote this book, my desire for sex ebbed and flowed as I learned more about each topic and myself. I used a lot of creative energy: reproductive, intellectual, editorial, and narrative. All that to say, my sex life was not as good as I wanted it to be in practice during this season, but I learned a lot that I can implement in the next season. That is a part of the grand point of this book.

I encourage you not to strive for perfect sex all the time. It's too much pressure. Further, you'll note that sexual frequency did not make the cut for the ingredients of good sex. It is more about quality than quantity, although nothing is wrong with either. I had many beautiful orgasms, more solo than partnered, to experience pleasure, inspire some creative thinking, and maintain my sexual well-being. And there are things I've written that my husband and I look forward to returning to during a slower paced, more intentional time in our life when we're not in the new baby twilight zone. I optimistically look forward to my own continued healing, learning, and sexual evolution. I look forward to doing "sexperiments" with myself and my husband, after we get through this postpartum period based on all that I learned and what I already know but just don't have the energy to implement yet. There is some good vacation sex coming our way to celebrate finishing this book, Love!

I am grateful that I get to be a sex scientist, though I wonder when the state of sex science will better reflect the lives of more than a narrow minority. When the education and training of mental health and medical professionals will better equip all of us to address good sex as an aspect of overall health.

I wonder how this book will be received, not for the desire to make the bestsellers lists and win awards, which I absolutely desire as an achievement-oriented person. But what is more important is if this will be a book that resonates with people who haven't really seen themselves in other sex books. Will the people who get left out benefit as much as, or more than, those who always have media catered to them? Will a precocious Black girl in her teens pick this book up, knowing good and well it wasn't written for her age group, and—like teenage me—try her best to piece together the sex education she wants and deserves that she can also share with her friends? I hope so.

Sexual liberation is an option for everyone, and every single person is worthy of it, but it will require psychological risk-taking to realize it. I want to be sure it's clear that good sex is worth the risk and the effort, but you also must know whether you have the room to make some of these changes. As you've noticed, some of the exercises take months, not just a moment. Rewriting your sexual menu isn't light work when so many systems of oppression have been organized around preventing people from experiencing good sex, for innumerable reasons. Try not to be too hard on yourself. If I, as a sex researcher and therapist who knows enough to write this book, am still working on making good sex a consistent practice in my life, then you are not alone in experiencing a few stalls. Just know that we can return to this practice at any time. Good sex is waiting on us, but there is a bunch of world changing and making that goes far beyond an individual trying exercises out for themselves.

The world I'm seeking to co-create, with my radical imagination and intentional action, is one where consent is core to our decision-making and relational style; where we don't set up our cultural recipes and systems to impose the values of a few people on as many people as possible; where we practice what we need to, rather than just talking a good talk, without external punishments and sanctions; and where our inherent sense of worthiness is honored.

As you select from this robust menu of good sex, I hope you join me in co-creating this world for yourself and others. That includes justice work to eliminate capitalism, overzealous religiosity, racism, sexism, heterosexism, ableism, ageism, ethnocentrism, and all the isms that fuck up good sex in your life and in the lives of people who have even more marginalization than you. Intimate justice is a viable and essential practice space for all of this. What you do with yourself and with your sexual partners has import in what occurs socially and politically. People who have established a healthy commitment to their own well-being, and good sex is absolutely a part of that, are better equipped to fuck these systems. That's what some people in power don't want you to know or realize.

I'm a better activist when I am taking good care of myself than when I'm not. I'm less of a hypocrite as a freedom fighter when I can assert the importance of erotic equity with my lover than when I don't. I resist better when I'm well rested and relaxed. My strategies for social justice are sounder when I am orgasming regularly. Maybe the same can be said for you.

ACKNOWLEDGMENTS

A foremother in sexology, Dr. June Dobbs Butts paved the way for me. In his outstanding thesis of her life, Je'lon Alexander details how Dr. Dobbs Butts was one of the first Black sexologists trained under Masters and Johnson. She became a professor, teaching and researching human sexuality for decades. She also maintained a robust community outreach practice, serving as a columnist for *Essence* and other leading magazines. Especially important to me, she was a Spelman alumna, as am I. There was so much overlap in our careers, and yet none of my training as a sexologist ever featured her. I didn't learn about her until her death in 2019. I am so grateful she had the courage to set the stage for someone like me, in a time where talking about sex was even more taboo.

Thank you to every therapy client and research participant who has shared their life with me. Thank you so much for entrusting me to journey with you. Thank you so much to Row House for believing in this book and to Tamela Julia Gordon and Lauren Alexander for editing it. Also, thank you to Theodore Burnes, Jessica Boyles, and Ayanay Ferguson for reading and providing feedback on early drafts. Thank you to Emily Nagoski, Laurie Mintz, Brittany Broaddus, Shamyra Howard, Goody Howard, and Debby Herbenick for reading and writing blurbs.

Thank you to everyone who has been a member of the RISE or RISE[2] Research Team for allowing me to be your academic mama. I appreciate the incredible work you've done on our research, and I would not be able to do this work without you: Louise Foster, Cynthia Doyle, Ixchel Collazo, Dashia Wright, Jaxin Annett, David Robinson, Carrie Bohmer, Anyoliny Sanchez, Queen-Ayanna Sullivan, Xinyue Lei, Caroline Adams, Hunter Savage, Jordan Brown, Brittany Cannon, Monyae Kerney, Rayven Peterson, Kascy Vigil, Courtney Wright, Destin Mizelle, Natalie Malone, Dr. Rena Curvey, Dr. Chesmore Montique, Dr. Jardin Dogan, Jennifer Stuck, Dr. Carolyn Meiller, Dr. Blanka Angyal, Dr. Brett Kirkpatrick, and Dr. Della V. Mosley.

I am grateful to my peer mentor turned colleague, sister friend, and work husband, Dr. Danelle Stevens-Watkins. Thank you for showing me the ropes in academia, being a true friend, and encouraging me to thrive.

I am grateful to my mentee turned colleague, sister friend, and academic auntie to my research kids, Dr. Shemeka Thorpe, who showed up at a time in my life where I had strayed from my love of sex research and helped me return to it.

Thank you also to all the Black women in sexology who helped Shemeka and I with the Big Sex Study: Tanya Bass, MEd, PhD, CHES, CSE; Robin Wilson-Beattie; M. Nicole Coleman, PhD; Yarneccia Dyson, PhD, MSW; Tracie Gilbert, PhD; Jasmine Johnson, MSW, MA, LCSW; Omisade Burney-Scott; and Marla Renee Stewart, MSW.

I am grateful to my late aunt Tonja Crowell who loved me unconditionally and showed me how fun it could be to be a hot girl.

Thank you to my parents, grandparents, siblings, extended family, and friends for believing I could do anything I set my mind to. I've always had a full bench of supporters and a lot of love because of you.

Last, but not least, thank you to my husband Ramon Hargons who gets to be my good sex practice partner for as long as we want to keep the beautiful vows we took. He who benefits from my sexual knowledge and suffers from my sexual shortcomings, loving me all the same, as I do with him.

Most importantly, I'm so grateful to sexual debut me, Candi Crowell, for being fast. I'm grateful to her for being curious, smart, driven, willing to fail, and ordering my steps to this moment of a dream come true. This book has been a long time coming, and I hope to keep coming.

BIBLIOGRAPHY

Alexander, Je'lon. "The Last Dame of the Dynasty: The Life and Legacy of Dr. June Dobbs Butts." Thesis, Georgia State University, 2021.

American Psychological Association. "Stress in America 2022." 2022.

Associated Press. "Methodist Church Approves Split of 261 Georgia Congregations after LGBTQ+ Divide." *Associated Press*, November 19, 2023.

Baleta, Adele. "Concern Voiced over 'Dry Sex' Practices in South Africa." *The Lancet* 352, no. 9136 (October 1998): 1292. https://doi.org/10.1016S0140 -6736(05)70507-9.

Barreto, Sydelle. "Fat and Forgotten: The Exclusion of Fat Women in Sexual Liberation and the Implications for Sexual Public Health." Thesis, The George Washington University, 2023.

Basson, Rosemary. "Human Sex-Response Cycles." *Journal of Sex & Marital Therapy* 27 no. 1 (2001): 33–43. https://doi.org/10.1080/00926230152035831.

Bienville, D. T. de. "Nymphomania, or a Dissertation Concerning the Furor Uterinus." Translated by E. S. Wilmot. London, 1775.

Birnie-Porter, Carolyn. "Intimacy and Sexual Relationships." *The Wiley Blackwell Encyclopedia of Gender and Sexuality Studies* (April 2016). https://doi. org/10.1002/9781118663219.wbegss628.

Braun, Virginia, Nicola Gavey, and Kathryn McPhillips. "The 'Fair Deal'? Unpacking Accounts of Reciprocity in Heterosex." *Sexualities* 6, no. 2 (May 2003): 237–61. https://doi.org/10.1177/1363460703006002005.

Brito Sena, Marina Aline de, Rodolfo Furlan Damiano, Giancarlo Lucchetti, and Mario Fernando Prieto Peres. "Defining Spirituality in Healthcare: A Systematic Review and Conceptual Framework." *Frontiers in Psychology* 12 (November 2021). https://doi.org/10.3389/fpsyg.2021.756080.

Brown, Adrienne Maree. *Pleasure Activism: The Politics of Feeling Good.* Chico, CA: AK Press, 2019.

Brown, Ashley, Edward D. Barker, and Qazi Rahman. "A Systematic Scoping Review of the Prevalence, Etiological, Psychological, and Interpersonal Factors Associated with BDSM." *The Journal of Sex Research* 57, no. 6 (October 2020): 781–811. https://doi.org/10.1080/00224499.2019.1665619.

Brown, Sherronda. *Refusing Compulsory Sexuality: A Black Asexual Lens on Our Sex-Obsessed Culture.* Berkeley: North Atlantic Books, 2022.

Busby, Dean M., Veronica Hanna-Walker, Nathan D. Leonhardt, and James J. Kim. "Sexual Passion in Couple Relationships: Emerging Patterns from Dyadic Response Surface Analysis." *Journal of Marriage and Family* 85, no. 1 (October 2022): 92–115. https://doi.org/10.1111/jomf.12888.

Carpenter, Deanna, Erick Janssen, Cynthia Graham, Harrie Vorst, and Jelte Wicherts. "Women's Scores on the Sexual Inhibition/Sexual Excitation Scales (SIS/SES): Gender Similarities and Differences." *Journal of Sex Research* 45, no. 1 (February 2008): 36–48. https://doi.org/10.1080/00224490701808076.

Cascalheira, Cory J., Ellen E. Ijebor, Yelena Salkowitz, Tracie L. Hitter, and Allison Boyce. "Curative Kink: Survivors of Early Abuse Transform Trauma through BDSM." *Sexual and Relationship Therapy* 38, no. 3 (2023): 353–83. https://doi.org/10.1080/14681994.2021.1937599.

Centers for Disease Control and Prevention. "Incidence, Prevalence, and Cost of Sexually Transmitted Infections in the United States, 2018." March 8, 2024.

Chadwick, Sara B., Miriam Francisco, and Sari M. van Anders. "When Orgasms Do Not Equal Pleasure: Accounts of 'Bad' Orgasm Experiences During Consensual Sexual Encounters." *Archives of Sexual Behavior* 48, no. 8 (September 2019): 2435–59. https://doi.org/10.1007/s10508-019-01527-7.

Clarke, Rebecca W., Chelom E. Leavitt, and Dean M. Busby. "Religious Piety and Sexual Passion: What Is the Connection?" *Journal of Sex & Marital Therapy* 48, no. 3 (2022): 221–37. https://doi.org/10.1080/0092623X.2021.1979702.

Crittenden, Patricia. "DMM Model." Accessed June 17, 2024. https://familyrelations institute.org/dmm-model/.

Darling, Carol Anderson, J. Kenneth Davidson, and Donna A. Jennings. "The Female Sexual Response Revisited: Understanding the Multiorgasmic Experience in Women." *Archives of Sexual Behavior* 20, no. 6 (1991): 527–40. https://doi.org/10.1007/BF01550952.

DeGue, Sarah, Linda Anne Valle, Melissa K. Holt, Greta M. Massetti, Jennifer L. Matjasko, and Andra Teten Tharp. "A Systematic Review of Primary Prevention

Strategies for Sexual Violence Perpetration." *Aggression and Violent Behavior* 19, no. 4 (July–August 2014): 346–62. https://doi.org/10.1016/j.avb.2014.05.004.

Diamond, Lisa M. and David M. Huebner. "Is Good Sex Good for You? Rethinking Sexuality and Health." *Social and Personality Psychology Compass* 6, no. 1 (January 2012): 54–69. https://doi.org/10.1111/j.1751-9004.2011.00408.x.

Division of HIV Prevention, National Center for HIV, Viral Hepatitis, STD, and TB Prevention, Centers for Disease Control and Prevention. "Pre-Exposure Prophylaxis (PrEP)." 2022.

DJ Simon Says. "Big Sex Playlist." N.d. https://open.spotify.com/playlist/6G0Kvz CYmkIeozaiekGQ4C?si=17944601e40a473f.

Dogan, Jardin N., Shemeka Y. Thorpe, Natalie Malone, Jasmine Jester, Danelle Stevens-Watkins, and Candice Hargons. "'My Partner Will Think I'm Weak or Overthinking My Pain': How Being Superwoman Inhibits Black Women's Sexual Pain Disclosure to Their Partners." *Culture, Health & Sexuality* 25, no. 5 (2023): 567–81. https://doi.org/10.1080/13691058.2022.2072956.

Edwards, D., and N. Panay. "Treating Vulvovaginal Atrophy/Genitourinary Syndrome of Menopause: How Important Is Vaginal Lubricant and Moisturizer Composition?" *Climacteric* 19, no. 2 (2016): 151–61. https://doi.org/10.3109 /13697137.2015.1124259.

Fahs, Breanne. "'Freedom to' and 'Freedom from': A New Vision for Sex-Positive Politics." *Sexualities* 17, no. 3 (May 2014): 267–90. https://doi.org/10.1177 /1363460713516334.

Fahs, Breanne, and Rebecca Plante. "On 'Good Sex' and Other Dangerous Ideas: Women Narrate Their Joyous and Happy Sexual Encounters." *Journal of Gender Studies* 26, no. 1 (2017): 33–44. https://doi.org/10.1080/09589236.2016.1246999.

Fogel Mersy, Lauren, and Jennifer Vencill. *Desire: An Inclusive Guide to Navigating Libido Differences in Relationships*. Boston: Beacon Press, 2023.

Frederick, David A., H. Kate St. John, Justin R. Garcia, and Elisabeth A. Lloyd. "Differences in Orgasm Frequency Among Gay, Lesbian, Bisexual, and Heterosexual Men and Women in a U.S. National Sample." *Archives of Sexual Behavior* 47 (2018): 273–88. https://doi.org/10.1007/s10508-017-0939-z.

Frederick, David A., Janet Lever, Brian Joseph Gillespie, and Justin R. Garcia. "What Keeps Passion Alive? Sexual Satisfaction Is Associated with Sexual Communication, Mood Setting, Sexual Variety, Oral Sex, Orgasm, and Sex Frequency in a National U.S. Study." *The Journal of Sex Research* 54, no. 2 (2017): 186–201. https://doi.org/10.1080/00224499.2015.1137854.

Gay & Lesbian Archives of the Pacific Northwest. "History of Sodomy Laws." April 15, 2007. https://www.glapn.org/sodomylaws/history/history.htm.

Granados, Reina, Joana Carvalho, and Juan Carlos Sierra. "Preliminary Evidence on How the Dual Control Model Predicts Female Sexual Response to a Bogus Negative Feedback." *Psychological Reports* 124, no. 2 (April 2021): 502–20. https://doi.org/10.1177/0033294120907310.

Greene, Kathryn, and Sandra L. Faulkner. "Gender, Belief in the Sexual Double Standard, and Sexual Talk in Heterosexual Dating Relationships." *Sex Roles* 53 (August 2005): 239–51. https://doi.org/10.1007/s11199-005-5682-6.

Groneman, Carol. *Nymphomania: A History.* New York: W. W. Norton & Company, 2000.

Gross, Neil. "The Detraditionalization of Intimacy Reconsidered." *Sociological Theory* 23, no. 3 (September 2005): 286–311. https://doi.org/10.1111/j.0735-2751.2005.00255.x.

Guttmacher Institute. "Sex and HIV Education." September 1, 2023. https://www.guttmacher.org/state-policy/explore/sex-and-hiv-education.

Hammond, Ashley S., Danielle F. Royer, and John G. Fleagle. "The Omo-Kibish I Pelvis." *Journal of Human Evolution* 108 (July 2017):199–219. https://doi.org/10.1016/j.jhevol.2017.04.004.

Handy, Ariel B., and Cindy M. Meston. "An Objective Measure of Vaginal Lubrication in Women With and Without Sexual Arousal Concerns." *Journal of Sex & Marital Therapy* 47 no. 1 (2021): 32–42. https://doi.org/10.1080/0092623X.2020.1801542.

Hargons, Candice N., Courtney J. Wright, Shemeka Thorpe, Destin L. Mizelle, Kasey Vigil, Hunter A. Savage, Jaxin Annett, Natalie Malone, and Rayven L. Peterson. "'It's What Boys Do': Valence, Source, and Content of Black Men's Masturbation Messages." Psychology of Men & Masculinities 25, no. 1 (2024): 33–43. https://doi.org/10.1037/men0000456.

Hargons, Candice N., Della Mosley, Carolyn Meiller, Jardin Dogan, Jennifer Stuck, Chesmore Montique, Natalie Malone, Carrie Bohmer, Queen-Ayanna Sullivan, Anyoliny Sanchez, et al. "'No One Can Make that Choice for You': Exploring Power in the Sexual Narratives of Black Collegians." *Journal of Counseling Sexology & Sexual Wellness: Research, Practice, and Education* 2, no. 2 (January 2020): 80–92. https://doi.org/10.34296/02021040.

Hargons, Candice N., Natalie Malone, Chesmore Montique, Jardin Dogan, Jennifer Stuck, Carolyn Meiller, Anyoliny Sanchez, Queen-Ayanna Sullivan, Carrie Bohmer R. Curvey, et al. "'White People Stress Me Out All the Time': Black Students Define Racial Trauma." *Cultural Diversity and Ethnic Minority Psychology* 28, no. 1 (2021): 49–57. https://doi.org/10.1037/cdp0000351.

Hargons, Candice N, Shemeka Thorpe, Natalie Malone, Courtney J Wright, Jardin N Dogan, Destin L Mizelle, Jennifer L Stuck, et al. 2024. "Black People's Constructions of Good Sex: Describing Good Sex from the Margins." *Sexualities* 27 (3): 457–74. https://doi.org/10.1177/13634607221101854.

Hatfield, Elaine, and Richard Rapson. *Love and Sex: Cross-Cultural Perspectives.* Boston: Allyn & Bacon, 1995.

Hepworth Clarke, Zelaika. "Osunality for Sexuality Educators, Clinicians, Researchers and Advocates." *The Journal of Sexual Medicine* 14, no. supplement_4b (May 2017): e273. https://doi.org/10.1016/j.jsxm.2017.04.321.

Herbenick, Debby, Heather Eastman-Mueller, Tsung-chieh Fu, Brian Dodge, Kia Ponander, and Stephanie A. Sanders. "Women's Sexual Satisfaction, Communication, and Reasons for (No Longer) Faking Orgasm: Findings from a U.S. Probability Sample." *Archives of Sexual Behavior* 48 (2019): 2461–72. https://doi.org/10.1007/s10508-019-01493-0.

Herz, Rachel S., and Elizabeth D. Cahill. "Differential Use of Sensory Information in Sexual Behavior as a Function of Gender." *Human Nature* 8 (1997): 275–86. https://doi.org/10.1007/BF02912495.

Higgins, Jenny A., Madison Lands, Mfonobong Ufot, and Sara I. McClelland. "Socioeconomics and Erotic Inequity: A Theoretical Overview and Narrative Review of Associations Between Poverty, Socioeconomic Conditions, and Sexual Wellbeing." *The Journal of Sex Research* 59, no. 8 (2022): 940–56. https://doi.org/10.1080/00224499.2022.2044990.

hooks, bell. *All About Love: New Visions.* New York: William Morrow, 1999.

Howard, Shamyra. *Use Your Mouth: Pocket-Sized Conversations to Simply Increase 7 Types of Intimacy in and out of the Bedroom.* Kindle, 2020.

Idelson-Shein, Iris. "Of Wombs and Words: Migrating Misogynies in Early Modern Medical Literature in Latin and Hebrew." *AJS Review: The Journal of the Association for Jewish Studies* 46, no. 2 (November 2022): 243–69. https://doi.org/10.1353/ajs.2022.0042.

Jamieson, Lynn. "Intimacy." *The Blackwell Encyclopedia of Sociology.* Wiley. February 2007. https://doi.org/10.1002/9781405165518.wbeosi071.

Janssen, Erick, Harrie Vorst, Peter Finn, and John Bancroft. "The Sexual Inhibition (SIS) and Sexual Excitation (SES) Scales: I. Measuring Sexual Inhibition and Excitation Proneness in Men." *The Journal of Sex Research* 39, no. 2 (2002): 114–26. https://doi.org/10.1080/00224490209552130.

Jet Setting Jasmine. "Fetish Survey." Accessed June 18, 2024. https://www.jsjlinks.com/fetish-survey.

Kennedy, Caitlin E., Ping Teresa Yeh, Jingjia Li, Lianne Gonsalves, and Manjulaa Narasimhan. "Lubricants for the Promotion of Sexual Health and Well-Being: A Systematic Review." *Sexual and Reproductive Health Matters* 29, no. 3 (2022). https://doi.org/10.1080/26410397.2022.2044198.

Kink Clinical Practice Guidelines Project. "Clinical Practice Guidelines for Working with People with Kink Interests." kinkguidelines.com, December 2019.

Koletić, Goran, Ivan Landripet, Azra Tafro, Luka Jurković, Goran Milas, and Aleksandar Štulhofer. "Religious Faith and Sexual Risk Taking among Adolescents and Emerging Adults: A Meta-Analytic Review." *Social Science & Medicine* 291 (December 2021): 114488. https://doi.org/10.1016/j.socscimed .2021.114488.

Labrecque, Frédérike, Audrey Potz, Émilie Larouche, and Christian C. Joyal. "What Is So Appealing about Being Spanked, Flogged, Dominated, or Restrained? Answers from Practitioners of Sexual Masochism/Submission." *The Journal of Sex Research* 58, no. 4 (2021): 409–23. https://doi.org/10.1080/00224499.2020 .1767025.

Láng, András, Erin B. Cooper, and Norbert Meskó. "The Relationship Between Dimensions of Adult Attachment and Motivation for Faking Orgasm in Women." *The Journal of Sex Research* 57, no. 3 (2020): 278–84. https://doi.org/10 .1080/00224499.2018.1525333.

Lapakko, David. "Communication Is 93% Nonverbal: An Urban Legend Proliferates." *Communication and Theater Association of Minnesota Journal* 34, no. 1 (2015): 7–19. http://dx.doi.org/10.56816/2471-0032.1000.

Leaf, Caroline. *Who Switched Off My Brain?: Controlling Toxic Thoughts and Emotions.* Nashville: Thomas Nelson Inc, 2009.

Leonhardt, Nathan D., Rebecca W. Clarke, and Chelom E. Leavitt. "Religiosity, Sexual Satisfaction, and Relationship Satisfaction: The Moderating Role of Sexual Mindfulness and Sexual Sanctification." *Journal of Sex & Marital Therapy* 49, no. 2 (2023): 155–71. https://doi.org/10.1080/0092623X.2022.2080132.

Levin, Roy J. "The Ins and Outs of Vaginal Lubrication." *Sexual and Relationship Therapy* 18, no. 4 (2003): 509–13. https://doi.org/10.1080/146819903100016 09859.

Lewis, Ruth, and Cicely Marston. "Oral Sex, Young People, and Gendered Narratives of Reciprocity." *The Journal of Sex Research* 53, no. 7 (2016): 776–87. https://doi.org /10.1080/00224499.2015.1117564.

Loulan, JoAnn. "Research on the Sex Practices of 1566 Lesbians and the Clinical Applications." *Women & Therapy* 7, no. 2–3 (1988): 221–34. https://doi.org/10.1300 /J015v07n02_18.

Mallory, Allen B. "Dimensions of Couples' Sexual Communication, Relationship Satisfaction, and Sexual Satisfaction: A Meta-Analysis." *Journal of Family Psychology* 36, no. 3 (2022): 358–71. https://doi.org/10.1037/fam0000946.

Mallory, Allen B., Amelia M. Stanton, and Ariel B. Handy. "Couples' Sexual Communication and Dimensions of Sexual Function: A Meta-Analysis." *The Journal of Sex Research* 56, no. 7 (2019): 882–98. https://doi.org/10.1080/00224499 .2019.1568375.

Malone, Natalie, Shemeka Thorpe, Jasmine K. Jester, Jardin N. Dogan, Danelle Stevens-Watkins, and Candice N. Hargons. "Pursuing Pleasure Despite Pain: A Mixed-Methods Investigation of Black Women's Responses to Sexual Pain and Coping." *Journal of Sex & Marital Therapy* 48, no. 6 (2022): 552–66. https://doi .org/10.1080/0092623X.2021.2012309.

Mayo Foundation for Medical Education and Research. "Compulsive Sexual Behavior." April 19, 2023. https://www.mayoclinic.org/diseases-conditions /compulsive-sexual-behavior/symptoms-causes/syc-20360434.

Mazzei, Patricia. "Criminal Investigation Roils Florida Republican Party." *The New York Times*, November 30, 2023.

McManus, I. C., and Adrian Furnham. "'Fun, Fun, Fun': Types of Fun, Attitudes to Fun, and Their Relation to Personality and Biographical Factors." *Psychology* 1, no. 3 (August 2010): 159–68. https://doi.org/10.4236/psych.2010.13021.

Meiller, Carolyn, and Candice N. Hargons. "'It's Happiness and Relief and Release': Exploring Masturbation Among Bisexual and Queer Women." *Journal of Counseling Sexology & Sexual Wellness: Research, Practice, and Education* 1, no. 1 (2019): 3–13. https://doi.org/10.34296/01011009.

Meston, Cindy M., and David M. Buss. "Why Humans Have Sex." *Archives of Sexual Behavior* 36 (August 2007): 477–507. https://doi.org/10.1007/s10508 -007-9175-2.

Mintz, Laurie. *Becoming Cliterate: Why Orgasm Equality Matters—And How to Get It.* New York: HarperOne, 2017.

Muise, Amy, Ulrich Schimmack, and Emily A. Impett. "Sexual Frequency Predicts Greater Well-Being, But More Is Not Always Better." *Social Psychological and Personality Science* 7, no. 4 (2016): 295–302. https://doi.org /10.1177/1948550615616462.

Muñoz-García, Laura Elvira, Carmen Gómez-Berrocal, and Juan Carlos Sierra. "Evaluating the Subjective Orgasm Experience Through Sexual Context, Gender, and Sexual Orientation." *Archives of Sexual Behavior* 52 (May 2023): 1479–91. https://doi.org/10.1007/s10508-022-02493-3.

Nagoski, Emily. *Come As You Are: Revised and Updated: The Surprising New Science That Will Transform Your Sex Life*. New York: Simon & Schuster, 2021.

National Institute on Drug Abuse. "Drugs, Brains, and Behavior: The Science of Addiction." July 2020. https://nida.nih.gov/publications/drugs-brains-behavior -science-addiction/drugs-brain.

O'Doherty, Tamara, and Kathleen Cherrington. "Commodified BDSM Services: Professional Dominatrices' Views on Their Work and Its Criminalization." *Archives of Sexual Behavior* 52, no. 3 (2023): 1285–98. https://doi.org/10.1007 /s10508-022-02490-6.

Office of Justice Programs. "Responding to Transgender Victims of Sexual Assault." Office for Victims of Crime, June 2014. https://ovc.ojp.gov/sites/g/files/xyckuh226 /files/pubs/forge/index.html.

Pailet, Xanet. *Living an Orgasmic Life: Heal Yourself and Awaken Your Pleasure*. Nashville: TMA Press, 2018.

Palacios, Santiago, Sarah Hood, Temitayo Abakah-Phillips, Nina Savania, and Michael Krychman. "A Randomized Trial on the Effectiveness and Safety of 5 Water-Based Personal Lubricants." *The Journal of Sexual Medicine* 20, no. 4 (April 2023): 498–506. https://doi.org/10.1093/jsxmed/qdad005.

Pascoal, Patrícia Monteiro, Isabel de Santa Bárbara Narciso, and Nuno Monteiro Pereira. "What Is Sexual Satisfaction? Thematic Analysis of Lay People's Definitions." *The Journal of Sex Research* 51, no. 1 (2014): 22–30. https://doi.org /10.1080/00224499.2013.815149.

Peasant, Courtney, Gilbert R. Parra, and Theresa M. Okwumabua. "Condom Negotiation: Findings and Future Directions." *The Journal of Sex Research* 52, no. 4 (2015): 470–83. https://doi.org/10.1080/00224499.2013.868861.

Perel, Esther. *Mating in Captivity: Unlocking Erotic Intelligence*. New York: Harper Paperbacks, 2007.

Perel, Esther, and Mary Alice Miller. "Why Eroticism Should Be Part of Your Self-Care Plan." Accessed June 18, 2024. https://www.estherperel.com/blog /eroticism-self-care-plan.

Quinn-Nilas, Christopher. "Relationship and Sexual Satisfaction: A Developmental Perspective on Bidirectionality." *Journal of Social and Personal Relationships* 37, no. 2 (2020): 624–46. https://doi.org/10.1177/0265407519876018.

Ratelle, Catherine F., Noémie Carbonneau, Robert J. Vallerand, and Geneviève Mageau. "Passion in the Romantic Sphere: A Look at Relational Outcomes." *Motivation and Emotion* 37 (2013): 106–20. https://doi.org/10.1007/s11031 -012-9286-5.

Rehman, Uzma S., Danielle Balan, Siobhan Sutherland, and Julia McNeil. "Understanding Barriers to Sexual Communication." *Journal of Social and Personal Relationships* 36, no. 9 (2019): 2605–23. https://doi.org/10.1177/0265407518794900.

Rubinsky, Valerie, and Angela Hosek. "'We Have to Get over It': Navigating Sex Talk Through the Lens of Sexual Communication Comfort and Sexual Self-Disclosure in LGBTQ Intimate Partnerships." *Sexuality & Culture* 24 (2020): 613–29. https://doi.org/10.1007/s12119-019-09652-0.

Ryan, Chris, and Rachel Kinder. "Sex, Tourism and Sex Tourism: Fulfilling Similar Needs?" *Tourism Management* 17, no. 7 (November 1996): 507–18. https://doi.org/10.1016/S0261-5177(96)00068-4.

Seal, Brooke N., and Cindy M. Meston. "The Impact of Body Awareness on Women's Sexual Health: A Comprehensive Review." *Sexual Medicine Reviews* 8, no. 2 (April 2020): 242–55. https://doi.org/10.1016/j.sxmr.2018.03.003.

Simon, William, and John H. Gagnon. "Sexual Scripts: Permanence and Change." *Archives of Sexual Behavior* 15 (1986): 97–120. https://doi.org/10.1007/BF01542219.

Simpson, Jeffry A., and Nickola C. Overall. "Partner Buffering of Attachment Insecurity." *Current Directions in Psychological Science* 23, no. 1 (2014): 54–59. https://doi.org/10.1177/0963721413510933.

Simpson, Jeffry A, and W Steven Rholes. "Adult Attachment, Stress, and Romantic Relationships." *Current Opinion in Psychology* 13 (February 2017):19–24. https://doi.org/10.1016/j.copsyc.2016.04.006.

Smithers, Gregory D. *Reclaiming Two-Spirits: Sexuality, Spiritual Renewal & Sovereignty in Native America.* Boston: Beacon Press, 2022.

Sprinkle, Annie, and Beth Stephens. "What Is Ecosex?" Accessed June 18, 2024. https://theecosexuals.ucsc.edu/ecosex/.

Sternberg, Robert J. "A Triangular Theory of Love." *Psychological Review* 93, no. 2 (1986): 119–35. https://doi.org/10.1037/0033-295X.93.2.119.

Tatkin, Stan. *Wired for Love: How Understanding Your Partner's Brain and Attachment Style Can Help You Defuse Conflict and Build a Secure Relationship.* Oakland: New Harbinger Publications, 2012.

Tee Noir. "Hypersexuality & the Perfect P*ssy Complex." YouTube, August 31, 2022.

Thorpe, Shemeka, Jardin Dogan-Dixon, Natalie Malone, and Kaylee A. Palomino. "'Just Be Strong and Keep Going': The Influence of Superwoman Schema on Black Women's Perceived Expectations of Coping with Sexual Pain." *Culture, Health & Sexuality* 26, no. 3 (2024): 346–61. https://doi.org/10.1080/13691058.2023.2210199.

Thorpe, Shemeka, Praise Iyiewuare, Samuella Ware, Natalie Malone, Jasmine K. Jester, Jardin N. Dogan, and Candice N. Hargons. "'Why Would I Talk to Them about Sex?': Exploring Patient-Provider Communication Among Black Women Experiencing Sexual Pain." *Qualitative Health Research* 32, no. 10 (2022): 1527–43. https://doi.org/10.1177/10497323221110091.

Thorpe, Shemeka, Rayven L. Peterson, Natalie Malone, M. Nicole Coleman, Jaxin Annett, and Candice N. Hargons. "From Sin to Sexual Self-Awareness: Black Women's Reflection on Lifetime Masturbation Messages." *Archives of Sexual Behavior* 52 (May 2023): 1403–15. https://doi.org/10.1007/s10508-022-02473-7.

Timmerman, Gayle M. "A Concept Analysis of Intimacy." *Issues in Mental Health Nursing* 12, no. 1 (1991): 19–30. https://doi.org/10.3109/01612849109058207.

Ueda, Peter, Catherine H. Mercer, Cyrus Ghaznavi, and Debby Herbenick. "Trends in Frequency of Sexual Activity and Number of Sexual Partners Among Adults Aged 18 to 44 Years in the US, 2000-2018." *JAMA Network Open* 3, no. 6 (2020): e203833. https://doi.org/10.1001/jamanetworkopen.2020.3833.

Vidal, Céline M., Christine S. Lane, Asfawossen Asrat, Dan N. Barfod, Darren F. Mark, Emma L. Tomlinson, Amdemichael Zafu Tadesse, Gezahegn Yirgu, Alan Deino, William Hutchison, et al. "Age of the Oldest Known Homo Sapiens from Eastern Africa." *Nature* 601 (2022): 579–83. https://doi.org/10.1038/s41586-021-04275-8.

Wade, Jeannette M., Helyne Frederick, Sharon Parker, Hannah Dillon, and Britney Williams. "A Black Feminist Examination of Sexual Liberation and Sexual Stereotypes: Perspectives from Black Female College Students." *Journal of Black Sexuality and Relationships* 9, no. 1–2 (Summer–Fall 2022): 19–41. https://doi.org/10.1353/bsr.2022.0011.

Werner, Marlene, Michèle Borgmann, and Ellen Laan. "Sexual Pleasure Matters—and How to Define and Assess It Too. A Conceptual Framework of Sexual Pleasure and the Sexual Response." *International Journal of Sexual Health* 35, no. 3 (2023): 313–40. https://doi.org/10.1080/19317611.2023.2212663.

Westlake, Bryce, and Isabella Mahan. "An International Survey of BDSM Practitioner Demographics: The Evolution of Purpose for, Participation in, and Engagement with, Kink Activities." *The Journal of Sex Research*, November 15, 2023, 1–19. https://doi.org/10.1080/00224499.2023.2273266.

Wibowo, Erik, and Richard J. Wassersug. "Multiple Orgasms in Men—What We Know So Far." *Sexual Medicine Reviews* 4, no. 2 (April 2016): 136–48. https://doi.org/10.1016/j.sxmr.2015.12.004.

INDEX

ABOUT THE AUTHOR

DR. CANDICE NICOLE HARGONS is a leading expert in sex research and an advocate for sexual health and liberation. As an award-winning psychologist and associate professor at Emory University's Rollins School of Public Health, Dr. Hargons has dedicated her fifteen-year career to empowering people to embrace their sexuality with self-awareness and a sense of inherent worthiness. Her work transcends academic boundaries, with her research and clinical experience informing her engaging writing and public speaking.

Dr. Hargons has been featured in *The New York Times*, *The Wall Street Journal*, HuffPost, *Essence*, and more, making complex topics in sex both accessible and relatable. When she's not recovering-perfectionist-Capricorn-level-busy with researching or teaching, you can find her enjoying a good book, eating a delicious meal, or spending quality time with her loved ones.